SpringerBriefs in Criminology

More information about this series at http://www.springer.com/series/10159

Sayantani Guin

Prison Inmates Living with HIV in India

Case Studies from Prisons in Maharashtra

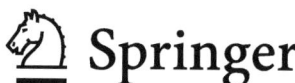 Springer

Sayantani Guin
School of Social Work
Indira Gandhi National Open University
New Delhi, India

ISSN 2192-8533   ISSN 2192-8541   (electronic)
SpringerBriefs in Criminology
ISBN 978-3-319-15565-4   ISBN 978-3-319-15566-1   (eBook)
DOI 10.1007/978-3-319-15566-1

Library of Congress Control Number: 2015931511

Springer Cham Heidelberg New York Dordrecht London

Printed on acid-free paper

Springer International Publishing AG Switzerland is part of Springer Science+Business Media
(www.springer.com)

Preface

This brief is based on a research study on the experiences of prison inmates living with HIV, conducted in three prisons in the state of Maharashtra, India. Based on seven case studies of prison inmates living with HIV, the author explores the health-care services in three prisons in Maharashtra, India, and highlights the major issues and problems faced by prison inmates living with HIV. The study also highlights the views and experiences of prison doctors and other prison staff vis-à-vis HIV in prisons. The results of the study aren't conclusive, but are hypotheses based on the study findings that raise questions and highlight areas for future research.

The study does not attempt to make broad conclusions about the state of HIV in prisons in India but rather sheds light on specific issues and opens up the area for further research. Attempt has been made to keep names of places and persons confidential. Mention of names of persons and places, if any, are meant purely for academic research purpose and not intended to malign the reputation of any person or institution.

The first chapter titled 'Introduction' explains the situation of HIV and the response to AIDS in prisons. This chapter is based on the review of various research studies conducted across the globe and in India on HIV in the prison setting. The chapter also presents the methodology of the present study, including the objectives, research setting, and tools employed, to conduct the research. Following a qualitative approach, the study adopted a multiple case study design to prepare detailed case studies of seven prison inmates living with HIV, through in-depth unstructured interview. The primary data are strengthened and substantiated by data collected from the prison medical officers and other prison staff through focus group discussions. Data were in the form of narratives, which were presented case wise. Qualitative analysis of the data was undertaken. The analysis process was geared towards describing and explaining the prisoner's experience of living with HIV, the way they perceive their situation in the prison vis-à-vis the health-care services, prison living conditions, etc.

The second chapter, 'HIV in Prisons', elaborately explains the concepts of HIV, its prevalence, and epidemiology in general and in prisons in particular, globally and in India. The chapter also throws light on various aspects of vulnerability of the prison population to HIV, viz. prison inmate as a key population at higher risk, high-risk behaviour prior to and during incarceration, HIV-related diseases, etc. This chapter also discusses the machineries and strategies to prevent HIV in prisons, globally and in India, and concludes with a human rights approach to HIV.

The third chapter is 'Profile of prison inmates living with HIV'. This chapter presents the seven case studies in detail and analyses the socio-economic profile of the prison inmates living with HIV, their incarceration history, high-risk behaviour prior to incarceration, etc. The analysis covering several dimensions of social and economic background of the inmate population revealed that majority of inmates were convicts, married, and in the age group of 25–40 years. The majority of the inmates living with HIV were engaged in high-risk sexual behaviour before imprisonment. The chapter also throws light on the source and extent of knowledge and information of prison inmates on HIV.

The fourth chapter on 'Experiences of prison inmates living with HIV' highlights the experiences of prison inmates living with HIV in terms of prison living conditions, risk behaviour during incarceration, prison medical services, and adherence to ethical issues. Results revealed that overcrowding and inadequate nutrition were major concerns for inmates living with HIV as these were leading to deterioration of their health. No support system was available inside the prisons to address the stress-related issues of inmates living with HIV. The prison hospital did not have provisions to cater to the treatment needs of inmates living with AIDS. Confidentiality regarding the HIV-positive status could not be maintained inside the prison.

The views of the prison medical staff and other prison personnel regarding the situation of HIV in prisons are presented in the fifth chapter titled 'Prison Personnel & HIV-Views and Experiences'. The chapter highlights the experiences and opinions of prison doctors and other prison staff on working pattern of staff, appointment, training on HIV, peer educators, reasons for HIV in prisons, etc., and presents the problems faced and suggestions offered by prison doctors and other staff. Prison doctors did not receive any training on HIV before they were appointed inside the prison. Lack of lab technician, insufficient number of prison medical doctors, and inadequate medical equipment and supplies within the prison were highlighted as the major shortcomings inside the prison.

Finally, the last chapter offers the summary and conclusion of the present study.

New Delhi, India   Sayantani Guin

Acknowledgements

I wish to acknowledge my indebtedness to a number of people who have encouraged me, directly or indirectly, in carrying out the research reported in this book.

To begin with, I owe my sincere thanks to Prof. Arvind Tiwari, who amongst all adversities guided my way forward leading to the completion of the research work. I thank the University Grants Commission, New Delhi, for providing me financial assistance in the form of JRF and SRF to complete the study. I wish to thank the Inspector General of Prisons, Maharashtra State, for granting permission during various stages of field work. I am particularly grateful to all the prison officials, the prison doctors, and the paramedical staff of the three prisons for their cooperation during the data collection. I wish to thank all the prison inmates who despite being unwell, very willingly participated in the research and made this study a success.

A special thanks to the Research Officer, Inspectorate of Prisons, Maharashtra, for making available the secondary data on prisons. I am also indebted to Deputy Director, National AIDS Research Institute, Pune, for sparing his valuable time for the interview. I am particularly thankful to the AIDS Nodal Officer and Secretary of Pune City AIDS Control Society, and the Additional Inspector General of Prisons, Hyderabad, for responding promptly to my queries and providing valuable information for the study.

My heartiest thanks go to all my friends and colleagues for their constant encouragement to complete the work.

I owe a great debt to my parents who have been a source of constant inspiration and always supported my dreams and aspirations. My sincere thanks go to my husband Prosanjit for his support and help in many ways to complete this book. I am grateful to my son Sattwik for his unconditional love and for showing me the greener side of life.

I am deeply indebted to Mr. Sumit Roy, the developmental editor, for painstakingly reading through the lines and cleaning up the manuscript within a very short period of time. His invaluable suggestions have strengthened the manuscript and constant encouragement has helped in finishing the project.

Last but not least, I would like to thank the anonymous reviewers and Springer editors for their comments and suggestions. A special thanks to Katie for her cooperation and support in finalizing the project.

November 2014   Sayantani Guin

Abbreviations

AIDS	Acquired Immunodeficiency Syndrome
ART	Antiretroviral Therapy
ARV	Antiretrovirals
BPR&D	Bureau of Police Research and Development
CMO	Chief Medical Officer
DIG	Deputy Inspector General
DOTS	Direct Observatory Treatment with Short Course Chemotherapy
ECG	Electrocardiogram
FGD	Focus Group Discussion
HIV	Human Immunodeficiency Virus
ICTC	Integrated Counselling and Testing Centre
IG	Inspector General of Prisons
MBBS	Bachelor of Medicine, Bachelor of Surgery
MCP	Mumbai Central Prison
MO	Medical Officer
MSM	Men who have sex with Men
NACO	National AIDS Control Organization
NACP	National AIDS Control Program
NARI	National AIDS Research Institute
NCRB	National Crime Records Bureau
NDPS	Narcotic Drugs and Psychotropic Substances
NGO	Non-Governmental Organization
NHRC	National Human Rights Commission
OPD	Outpatient Department
STD	Sexually Transmitted Disease
STI	Sexually Transmitted Infection
TB	Tuberculosis
UNAIDS	United Nations Program on HIV and AIDS
UNGASS	United Nations General Assembly Special Session

UNODC	United Nations Office on Drugs and Crime
USAIDS	United States Agency for International Development
UT	Union Territory
VCTC	Voluntary Counselling and Testing Centre
WHO	World Health Organization

Contents

About the Author

Sayantani Guin is Assistant Professor of Social Work at the School of Social Work in Indira Gandhi National Open University (IGNOU), New Delhi. She holds Ph.D. and M.Phil. degrees in Social Sciences from Tata Institute of Social Sciences (TISS), Mumbai. She has a Master's degree in Social Work with specialization in Criminology and Correctional Administration from TISS. She has presented various academic and research papers at several International and National Conferences held in India and abroad. She has published extensively in a wide range of international scholarly journals. Her academic and research interests include Social Work, Administration of Criminal Justice, and HIV and AIDS in prisons.

Chapter 1
Introduction

The HIV epidemic has drawn attention to the existing health-care services of many prison systems around the world. The study of prison inmates living with HIV is not only complex and critical but also deals with a sensitive issue. Addressing the basic HIV-related health-care concerns inside the prison, viz. HIV prevention, HIV-related diseases, AIDS diagnosis, prison medical services, etc., usually meets with various administrative barriers. The spread of HIV within the prison premises, mainly through injecting drug use and homosexual activity, is either ignored or meets with disciplinary measures (Jurgens 2007).

Prisoners are often the forgotten lot of the society. Many of them belong to the marginalized and disadvantaged sections of the general population. They might be urban poor, minorities, immigrants, or Injecting Drug Users, who had limited or no access to basic medical care. They might have also been subjected to malnutrition, illiteracy, unhealthy living condition, unemployment, etc. When these people are imprisoned due to their criminal status, their life is jeopardized further by the deplorable prison conditions characterized by overcrowding, poor hygiene, inadequate nutrition, and lack of ventilation (Goyer 2003).

Access to basic health care inside the prison is limited because of many factors like lack of medical facilities, inadequate staff, insufficient funding of health services, etc. Thus, the deplorable conditions coupled with lack of health-care services makes the prison breeding ground for different types of infections. This has a greater impact on the life span of a prison inmate living with HIV, which might in the extreme scenario lead to death (Goyer 2003).

The State restrains criminals of certain rights and liberties through imprisonment because of the crimes they commit. However, exposing them to fatal diseases is not only inhuman but also a violation of the human rights of the inmates. It, then, turns into a double sentence for the criminal. Various international treaties and covenants confer the right to health care and right not to contract disease inside the prison. Many International instruments, specifically International Guidelines on HIV/AIDS and Human Rights, 1996, United Nations General Assembly Special Session on

© The Author(s) 2015
S. Guin, *Prison Inmates Living with HIV in India,*
SpringerBriefs in Criminology, DOI 10.1007/978-3-319-15566-1_1

HIV/AIDS (UNGASS), June 2001, and The World Health Organization (WHO) Guidelines on HIV Infection and AIDS in Prisons, 1993, are relevant to the condition of prisoners, in the context of HIV. International guidelines advocate the 'equivalence principle' or the idea that the same care should be provided in prisons that is available to the general public (Goyer 2003).

A criminal faces imprisonment either as an undertrial or as a convict. It is all the more important to control any contagious disease within the prison premises, so as to ensure that it does not spread in the community, once the prisoner is released back to the civil society. Further, it is imperative to address specific health concerns related to HIV, like TB and STI, in the community as it might aggravate the situation of HIV in prison, when a person is imprisoned (Goyer 2003).

This subject itself makes this study very significant, since the issue of a prison inmate living with HIV has not been much pursued in India, as compared to other parts of the world. This study focuses primarily on the experiences of prison inmates living with HIV in three prisons in the state of Maharashtra, India.

Review of Literature

Although most of the available literature on HIV in prisons has been developed by organizations like the United Nations Program on HIV/AIDS (UNAIDS), World Health Organization (WHO), United Nations Office on Drugs and Crime (UNODC), United States Agency for International Development (USAIDS), National AIDS Control Organization (NACO) etc., a few other agencies and individuals have also carried out studies on HIV in prisons, which have been published in the form of books, articles, monographs, and research studies.

For the purpose of analysis, in the review of literature, the different research studies have been divided into subheadings. These subheadings basically highlight the various aspects/issues that the existing research studies on HIV in prisons have captured, globally as well as in the Indian context. The findings of these studies have not only helped the researcher to understand the national and international scenario with regard to HIV in prisons but also played an important role in planning and designing the present study.

HIV Prevalence in Prison

Several research studies across the world indicate the prevalence of HIV in prison. While some studies indicate low prevalence (Sundar et al. 1995[1]; Dolan & Larney 2010[2]), others reveal high prevalence of HIV in prison (Singh 2008; Oppong et al.

---

[1] Twenty (1.98 %) undertrials out of 1,007 undertrials in Central Prison, Bangalore, India, were seropositive for HIV infection.

[2] 1.7 % prison inmates were HIV positive in India.

2013). The HIV prevalence in Armenian prison was 27 times higher than that in the general population (Weilandt et al. 2007). The overall HIV prevalence in Iranian prison was 2.8 %, which was more than that in the general population (around 0.1 %) (Haghdoost et al. 2013). Blogg et al. (2014) reported that HIV prevalence among prison inmates in Indonesia was 1.1 % among male and 6 % among female inmates. HIV prevalence varied from 0 to 13.2 % in different prisons in Iran (Haghdoost et al. 2013). Pal et al. (1999) carried out seroprevalence study of HIV infection among jail inmates in three prisons in Orissa, India, from March 1994 to December 1995. The study revealed that all the prisoners of Indian origin (300), housed in these jails, tested negative for HIV infection, while 33.8 % of jail inmates from foreign countries (Thailand & Myanmar), serving short terms in these jails of Orissa, were found to be HIV positive.

Profile of Prison Inmates Living with HIV

Studies reveal that prison inmates living with HIV have low literacy, poor income, sexual promiscuity, and low condom usage (Sundar et al. 1995). The male young inmates had higher risk of HIV infection, as compared to older female inmates (Swartz et al. 2004). Asl et al. (2013) reported that the mean age of prison inmates living with HIV was 31.4 years. Kalantar & Alijev (2005) noted that the average age of HIV-infected prisoners was 20–25 years. 14 % inmates were illiterate and 21 % had graduated from high school or attended university. 11 % of the participants reported being unemployed at the time of their incarceration. Fifty percent were single and had never been married, and of those who were married, 65 % had children (Asl et al. 2013).

High-Risk Behaviour During Incarceration

Research suggests that prison inmates engage in high-risk behaviour during incarceration and get exposed to HIV. High-risk behaviour during incarceration includes homosexual activity (Dolan & Larney 2010; Simooya & Sanjobo 2001), the use of contaminated injecting equipment for intravenous drug use, the use of contaminated cutting instruments for tattooing and piercing (Blogg et al. 2014), gang activity involving violence and victimization of younger inmates (Goyer 2003; Braithwaite et al. 1996; Weilandt et al. 2007; Krebs 2002; Singh 2008), inserting genital accessories without sterile equipment, and sex without condoms (Blogg et al. 2014). Chakrapani et al. (2013) reported availability of alcohol and injectable or oral drugs such as heroin, dextropropoxyphene, and marijuana inside prisons. Ray (2002) highlighted the various issues concerning drug abuse among the prisoners, over 4 years (1997–2000), as seen in Tihar Jail, New Delhi, India. The study aimed to provide understanding of the issues relating to drug abuse within the prison population. It studied the extent and pattern of drug abuse in a large prison of the country and described the profile of the drug abusers. The major components of this study were National Household Survey, Drug Abuse Monitoring System, and Rapid Assessment Survey. It stressed the fact that the data on drug abuse among prison population in India were virtually absent, though it was widely believed that a significant percentage of population in the prison might be addicted to one or more drugs. Highlighting the details of the prisoners' socio-economic background, the study took into consideration the treatment facilities and the monitoring mechanisms for drug users in Tihar Jail. The study recommended designing specific instruments to measure the quality of care provided for drug abusers in prisons and developing a monitoring instrument for prison population by setting up detoxification and rehabilitation centres in prisons in India. The study also recommended the use of therapeutic community model in prisons nationwide and extending treatment services to a larger number of prisoners under the NDPS Act.

Knowledge Regarding HIV

Some studies have tried to identify a correlation between knowledge on transmission and prevention of HIV and attitude towards people living with HIV. It is argued that poor knowledge was associated with negative attitude towards persons living with HIV (Weilandt et al. 2007). Knowledge regarding HIV was found to be superficial by Singh (2008), and poor knowledge on the transmission and prevention of infectious diseases was reported by Weilandt et al. (2007) in case of both the prisoners as well as the prison staff. A study by Swartz et al. (2004), however, suggested that despite knowledge, a substantial number of participants expressed willingness to participate in high-risk behaviours, such as unprotected sex with multiple partners and needle sharing, and, thus, were at high risk of HIV exposure. Kalantar & Alijev (2005) reported that the lack of knowledge about hygiene and the perils of HIV and other sexually transmitted diseases among prisoners contributed to new cases of HIV in prisons, every week.

Cause of High-Risk Behaviour

A number of studies have been conducted to identify the causes of high-risk behaviour among inmates. Some of the researchers have associated high-risk behaviour with high level of substance use prior to incarceration (Sifunda et al. 2007) or childhood sexual abuse (Mullings et al. 2003). Goyer (2003) reported that the socio-economic factors of the young, unemployed, undereducated black men that encouraged them into criminal activity and incarceration also led them to engage in high-risk behaviours, thereby making them prone to contract HIV. Weilandt et al. (2007) indicated that drug use in the prisons had a correlation to high-risk behaviour, although the rate of high-risk behaviour related to drug use in the prisons was quite low. Gillespie (2005) reported that those inmates, who were drug users before being incarcerated, had a propensity for drug abuse even after imprisonment. The study further concluded that the general factors positively associated with drug abuse among inmates were age (youth), race (white), prior habit of selling drugs on streets, and rule defying attitude. Moreover, those inmates who had served more years in prison, never participated in prison religious services, or had rule violating friends, were inclined towards drug abuse.

HIV Preventive Measures in Prison

Research studies have suggested various measures for the prevention of HIV transmission inside prisons. Many studies advocated for HIV education and information programmes, distribution of condoms, lubricants, and bleach, and/or needle exchange programmes (Goyer 2003; Weilandt et al. 2007). A study by West (2001) suggested that effective HIV prevention programmes should take into consideration the traditional Latin culture and gender roles, which prevented Latina women to negotiate condom use by their partners. A statistically significant increase in knowledge was observed after conducting HIV workshops among adult female inmates in the AIDS Counselling and Education (ACE) Program at Bedford Hills Correctional Facility in New York State. The workshops aimed to provide individual counselling, HIV testing, outreach services, support groups, annual events, professional trainings, discharge planning/case management, and effective follow-up services when the women were released, and catered annually to approximately 6,000 women inmates (Collica 2002). A race and gender-sensitive, peer-facilitated, multimedia HIV and Hepatitis protocol was developed to address HIV risk reduction and prevention for the re-entry population (Inciardi et al. 2007). A high-level intervention for HIV prevention and support service was available to approximately 70,000 inmates housed in 69 correctional facilities across New York State, in the form of HIV prevention education, individual and group counselling, and HIV support groups (Klein et al. 2002). A prison-based HIV intervention was most successful at influencing beliefs and response related to peer behaviour and somewhat successful at influencing beliefs and intentions related to condom use (Bryan et al. 2006). Sifunda et al. (2008) argued that peer-led health education programmes might be effective in reducing risky behaviour amongst soon-to-be-released inmates. Some studies (Simooya & Sanjobo 2001; Grinstead et al. 1999) highlighted the importance of peer educators, while others (Grinstead et al. 1999) stressed on the need for collaboration among academic research institutions, community-based organizations, prison staff, and inmate peer educators.

Problems Inside Prison: Systems and Conditions

Many researchers have focused on the problems faced by prison inmates living with HIV. The problem of overcrowding (Goyer 2003; Tiwari 2002; Singh 2008), stress, and malnutrition (Goyer 2003) were reported as compromising factors, worsening the overall health of all inmates, and particularly those living with HIV. Limited resources and ensuring adherence to treatment programmes were reported as some of the biggest challenges (Goyer 2003). Braithwaite et al. (1996) reported lack of access to condoms among inmates. Shalihu et al. (2014) reported six barriers to HIV antiretroviral therapy adherence among prison inmates living with HIV in Namibia—the need to maintain anonymity (because of the deep-rooted social stigma towards HIV), non-availability of basic resources for adherence (like a watch/clock to maintain timely intake of scheduled drugs), lack of nutrition to complement the taxing ART, commodification of ART medication, discouragement as a result of the awful prison conditions, and lack of awareness. Tiwari (2002) reported appalling conditions of overcrowding, lack of sanitation, inadequate diet, unhygienic living conditions, and lack of health awareness among prisoners as contributing factors for many diseases like tuberculosis, diarrhoea, anaemia, malarial fevers, skin diseases, sexually transmitted diseases, and respiratory problems. Singh (2008) reported superficial understanding of HIV among prison inmates, high prevalence of HIV in prison, and inadequate access to antiretroviral treatment. Some studies also revealed corruption (Tiwari 2002; Singh 2008) and inappropriate living conditions (Singh 2008) within prison. Somasundaram & Sundar (1997), in their article titled, 'Aiding AIDS Prisoners: Issues and Options', raised certain inherent difficulties associated with HIV & AIDS in a correctional setting and strived for the need for a separate set of rules for prisoners infected with HIV. Their literature review of various studies conducted abroad regarding the prevalence of HIV & AIDS in prisons highlighted that the prevalence rate of HIV & AIDS and that of diseases like tuberculosis is higher in prison populations as compared to the general populations. Apart from the prevalence rate, the studies conducted abroad also highlighted the screening options, costs involved in screening inmates, and issues concerning the management of prison inmates. This article raised various issues pertaining to dealing with prisoners living with HIV in prisons, viz. the need for epidemiological studies on HIV & AIDS in correctional institutions, Mandatory Testing vs. Optional Testing, Confidentiality vs. Disclosure and Segregation vs. Mainstreaming, etc. The authors suggested that among other things, the rules for dealing with prisoners living with HIV and AIDS should include HIV Testing, Confidentiality, Counselling, Medical attention and psycho-social services, accommodation and correctional management, anti-discriminatory provisions, special provisions for persons living with AIDS, research and information, education, and communication.

Addressing Ethical Issues

Studies suggest that mandatory HIV testing and segregation based on HIV-positive status are not supported internationally (Goyer 2003).

Post-Release Care

Some studies have focused on the continuity of care for prison inmates living with HIV, post-release from prison. Laufer et al. (2002) demonstrated the strategy of collaboration between public health department, jail facilities, and community-based organizations (CBO). This enabled the inmates to access HIV care and treatment not only while serving their terms, but even when they went back to their communities, after being released.

The Present Study

From the above, it may be said that there have been some efforts from the government and non-governmental organizations to address the situation of HIV in prisons. However, as evident, all these efforts have been piecemeal without any concrete and regular action being taken by the prison department to address the issue of HIV in prisons. Thus, it seems that HIV in prisons is being left out both by the Government machineries as well as by the non-governmental organizations.

As observed from the above literature review, it appears that a number of studies have been conducted in Indian prisons from time to time. However, most of these studies were confined to describing the appalling conditions of the prisons and other prison-related issues such as vocational training, education of prisoners, etc.

The rationale for the present study essentially emerged from the review of the available literature in the area of HIV in prisons in India. It was evident that very few studies were conducted on HIV in prisons, particularly in the Indian context. Except for the study in Tihar Jail, no comprehensive study was reported on problems of prisoners living with HIV in India. There was a gap in the existing literature on this issue, and thus, it became imperative to conduct this study. HIV in prisons is a worldwide phenomenon and India is no exception to it.

Prison population has always been a neglected lot when we consider issues of health in general and HIV in particular. The various studies that have been conducted over time on various aspects of the prison life in India have repeatedly documented about overcrowding, work and vocational training, lack of infrastructure, role of prison personnel in correctional activities, and plight of the children of women prisoners in Indian jails (Haikerwal 1939; Srivastava 1977; Khan 1990; Bedi 2002; Shankardass 2000; Chattoraj 2006). Very few studies have examined the state of health and medical facilities in prison setting (Srivastava 1977; Bedi 2002; Sarangi 1999; Tiwari 2002).

From the review of the literature, it was clear that more studies were necessary to elicit data required to explain the experiences of prison inmates living with HIV and the means to redress their problems.

The prison population consists of people regularly moving in and out. Whereas most prisoners, when released after completion of their term, directly move back into the community for good, some turn out to be habitual offenders and are imprisoned and released a number of times.

The present study explores the experiences of prison inmates living with HIV. It also attempts to understand the extent and quality of health care in jails on HIV care and prevention.

Objectives of the Study

The objectives of the present study are the following:

1. To examine the case history of the prison inmates living with HIV.
2. To provide an in-depth analysis of the situation in which they live in prison.
3. To understand the perception of prisoners (living with HIV), other prison inmates, prison personnel, and doctors (prison medical doctors and paramedical staff) regarding the health-care system in the prisons.
4. To suggest ways and means to resolve the problems faced by prison inmates living with HIV.

Research Design

This study is based on exploratory research design, to create an information base about the severity and seriousness of the HIV scenario in jails, which will guide further research on the issue.

Study Sites

Profile of Maharashtra

The state of Maharashtra, located on the west coast of India, is India's second largest state in terms of population with 9.29 % share of the country's total population and the third largest in terms of area. In terms of growth rate, Maharashtra ranks 21 in the country (Table 1.1).

Table 1.1 State profile—Maharashtra

Population	112,374,333
Males	58,243,056
Females	54,131,277
Sex ratio (females per 1,000 males)	929
Density of population (persons/sq.km)	365
Literacy rate (in percent)	82.34
Male literacy in (in per cent)	88.38
Female literacy in (in per cent)	75.87

Source: Census of India (2011)

Prisons in Maharashtra

Prison administration in India is a State subject. Prison establishments in the states/ union territories (UTs) comprise of several tiers of jails. The most common and standard jail institutions are known as Central Jails, District Jails, and Sub-Jails. The other types of jail institutions are Women Jails,[3] Borstal Schools,[4] Open Jails,[5] and Special Jails[6] (National Crime Records Bureau 2012).

The total number of prisons in the state of Maharashtra is 215, which includes nine Central Jails, 25 district prisons, 172 sub-jails, one women jail, one Borstal school, five open jails, and two special jails. The officially approved accommodation in these jails is 24,656 prisoners whereas the total inmate population is 24,509. Though the number of inmates is less than the official sanctioned accommodation, the Central Jails and the District Jails are all overcrowded. In Maharashtra, 32.7 % of the prison inmates are convicts and 67 % are undertrials (National Crime Records Bureau 2012).

---

[3] Women jails are prisons meant exclusively for women offenders.

[4] Borstal Schools are a type of youth detention centre and are used exclusively for the imprisonment of minors or juveniles. The primary objective of Borstal Schools is to ensure care, welfare, and rehabilitation of young offenders in an environment suitable for children and keep them away from disturbing atmosphere of the prison. The juveniles in conflict with law detained in Borstal Schools are provided vocational training and educational support with the help of trained teachers. The emphasis is given on the education, training, and moral influence conducive for their reformation and prevention of crime.

[5] An open jail is a unique kind of arrangement where the prisoners are kept under minimum security and vigil. However, only those prisoners who exhibit acceptable behaviour over a period of time, which adheres to certain prescribed guidelines, are eligible for open prisons.

[6] Special jails are meant for prisoners who are either convicted of highly heinous crimes, are habitual offenders, or exhibit highly unacceptable behaviour on a regular basis even within the jail. The security level is very high in these special jails as compared to other prisons.

The Three Prisons Under Study

The study was conducted in three central prisons in the districts of Mumbai, Pune, and Nasik, viz. Mumbai Central Prison, Yerwada Central Prison, and Nasik Road Central Prison in the state of Maharashtra. Maharashtra has the highest number (215) of prisons among the states/UTs in India (National Crime Records Bureau 2012). Official written permission was granted by the Inspector General of Prisons, Maharashtra, to collect the data, including review of inmate medical records.

Yerwada Central Jail

Yerwada Central Jail, established in the year 1871, is the largest jail in the state of Maharashtra, situated in the Western Region of the state. It is spread over 512 acres of land (Shaikh 2010), comprising various barracks and security zones, besides an open jail just outside its premises. It houses the highest number of convict prisoners. Many famous personalities like Mahatma Gandhi were imprisoned here, during the Indian independence movement in 1930s and 1940s. As of 31.12.2011, it housed 3,378 inmates in a sanctioned capacity of 2,449 (National Crime Records Bureau 2012).

Mumbai Central Jail

Mumbai Central Jail, popularly known as Arthur Road Jail, was built in 1926 and is Mumbai's largest and oldest prison. The jail is spread over 2 acres of land. It was built by the British rulers of India as a transit prison and was situated outside the then city limits. Over the years, however, the city has engulfed the prison and the high-security facility is now surrounded by residential and commercial establishments (Plumber & Pathak 2011). It houses 2,162 prisoners in a sanctioned capacity of 804 (National Crime Records Bureau 2012). It is situated in the southern region of Maharashtra and houses the highest number of undertrials in the state.

Nasik Road Central Jail

Nasik Road Central Jail was established in the year 1927 (Inspector General of Prisons 2006). The total sanctioned capacity of the jail was 3,178 and the number of inmates was 2,151 (National Crime Records Bureau 2012). The prison has 113 acres of agricultural land within its premises and five of the ten existing wells are being used for agricultural purposes. Over 50 % of the agricultural land is not being utilized (Sonawane 2014). It is situated in the central region of Maharashtra.

Tools of Data Collection

Primary data were collected through in-depth interviews, guided by Interview Guide. Data were gathered to access information from the prisoners living with HIV, prisoners not affected by HIV, prison personnel, prison doctors, and para-medical staff. However, since permission for using tape recorder inside the jail was denied, the researcher had to write down the major pointers and specific comments.

In each of the three jails, one Focus Group Discussion (FGD) was conducted with each of the five groups—prisoners living with HIV, prisoners not affected by HIV, prison personnel, prison doctors, and paramedical staff. Each FGD was con-ducted with an average number of four to eight participants. The researcher initiated each Group Discussion and then facilitated it, allowing interactive discussions. The data gathered through FGDs were categorized into themes. The major themes focused on access to health-care services for inmates living with HIV, management of STIs and other infectious diseases and chronic conditions, health care-seeking behaviour, referral systems, and provision of facility-based health interventions for inmates in general and inmates living with HIV in particular.

Pilot visits were made in each of the three prisons to frame the interview ques-tions. The medical officer of each prison was consulted to help identify the prison inmates living with HIV. Three prison inmates living with HIV were interviewed one-on-one, one in each of the pilot visits. Three case studies were prepared from the narratives of these inmates. Qualitative analysis of the data was undertaken to capture the way the inmates living with HIV perceive health-care services in prison. This analysis helped to identify issues, themes, and content for framing the interview guides. The in-depth interviews were conducted using a semi-structured interview guide. The semi-structured interview guide was developed based on the data gathered through pilot visits and the available literature on health services in correctional institutions. Most of the themes explored were chosen to ensure that interviews elicited meaningful information on correctional health issues, especially with respect to HIV. The major themes focused on access to health-care services for inmates living with HIV, management of infectious diseases and chronic condi-tions, health care-seeking behaviour, referral systems, and provision of facility-based health interventions for inmates in general and inmates living with HIV in particular.

Procedures

The researcher had to take necessary approvals before beginning the study. The proposal was presented before a Board responsible for granting approvals of research studies. All the ethical issues regarding confidentiality, informed consent, etc., were raised and clarified to the board. It was only when the board got convinced with all the issues that the study was approved. Moreover, before proceeding for data collection, permission for data collection was also sought from the Inspector General of Prisons, Maharashtra state.

Participants

Reported cases of HIV-positive male inmates were selected for the study and were used as the unit of analysis.

In the pilot study, the researcher ascertained the number of reported HIV-positive inmates in each prison, which was negligible compared to the total number of inmates in each of the prisons. Initially, the total number of HIV-positive inmates to be interviewed was not fixed and data were collected until there was saturation in data. The prison medical officer helped in identifying the HIV-positive inmates and shared their medical reports with the researcher. Interviews were conducted in a room adjacent to that of the prison medical doctor. Apart from the doctor and the medical helper (who handled the medical records and hence already knew the HIV-positive status of the inmates), it was ensured that no one else could know about the interview, thus maintaining confidentiality. In addition, the interview was not audible to the medical officer as he was in a different room. Before beginning the interview, the researcher introduced herself to the respondent and explained the purpose of the research. Only those inmates who gave verbal consent for the interview were interviewed. One-on-one, semi-structured in-depth interviews were conducted with seven HIV-positive inmates. The interviews were conducted in Hindi, the most widely spoken language in India. All of the participants understood and spoke Hindi. The duration of each interview was around 20–30 minutes. Field notes were used to gather data during the interviews. Subsequently, case studies of the seven inmates were prepared based on their narratives. No payment was offered or made and the participation of each respondent was voluntary.

Qualitative analysis of the data was geared towards describing and explaining inmates' experience of living with HIV in prison. Data collected through the interviews were coded into major themes. During coding, emerging themes and patterns were constantly added.

Ethical Considerations

HIV being a very sensitive issue, the following ethical considerations were adhered to:

Informed Consent

While seeking a respondent's participation in the study and before the interview, the researcher clearly informed the prospective participant in detail, the factors such as the risks and benefits that the research may expose the participant to, the absence of monetary or material inducement, the purpose of the research, the academic institution the researcher belonged to, duties and responsibilities of the researcher, the manner of keeping records, and the guarantee of confidentiality. The respondents were convinced that their name would not be mentioned in the study. This discussion was followed by the researcher asking the inmate's willingness to participate. The prisoners were interviewed only after their voluntary verbal consent to participate.

Confidentiality

No information relating to inmate's identity, such as the name or address, has been revealed. This has been done to protect the interest of the prisoner and keep his HIV-positive status confidential.

Limitations of the Study

Before entry into the prisons for data collection, the researcher had to do a lot of initial homework. The research setting being a closed structured setting unlike the usual open field settings, permission had to be sought from the Inspector General of Prisons, Maharashtra, during the research proposal writing stage itself. A request letter, elaborately describing the research objectives and scope of study, was sent to the Inspector General of Prisons, Maharashtra, in order to get permission for data collection. The request letter was written on behalf of the research guide and not on behalf of the researcher, to ensure that permission was granted promptly. However, permission was not granted at the very first instance and the researcher was asked to prove her nationality by the Inspector General of Prisons, Maharashtra. Once the researcher submitted the documents to prove her nationality, she was permitted to collect data from the three jails. However, the visits in the prisons were dependent on the availability and the suitability of the prison officials. Before each visit to the jail, the researcher had to formally inform the respective Prison Superintendent about her visit and request him to make the necessary arrangements. At many instances, despite having prior permission, the researcher had to wait at the prison gate, before being permitted inside by the Superintendent. A major limitation faced by the researcher was the limited access inside the jail for conducting the interviews with the prisoners, due to security reasons. The inmates expressed their expectation from the researcher from time to time during the interview, by requesting the intervention of the researcher in either matters related to their disease or administrative issues like jail transfer. At such instances, the researcher had to apologize and admit her limitations as a researcher.

Chapter 2
HIV in Prisons

HIV or Human Immunodeficiency Virus has not only posed a major challenge to modern medical science but has also emerged as a serious public health concern. On one hand, the virus eventually leads to AIDS due to lack of any medicine; on the other hand, it is often associated with a lot of stigma, prejudice, fear, and silence. The social denial (of incidence of HIV) and lack of knowledge and awareness regarding the virus often contribute to neglect of care and treatment for people living with HIV (Goyer 2003).

The situation of HIV in the prisons is an issue which is often ignored and neglected. This is mainly because of the fact that prisoners are often the forgotten lot of the society. Coupled with the stigma associated with HIV, prison inmates are often doubly victimized in terms of access to care and treatment (Goyer 2003).

Several issues need to be considered with regard to HIV in prison setting. Prison inmates are at risk of contracting HIV because they engage in high-risk behaviour, viz. homosexuality, use of non-sterile contaminated injecting equipments, tattooing, etc. The risk is aggravated by the prison conditions characterized by overcrowding, boredom, inadequate access to health services, etc. Prison inmates, being a floating population, may infect partners, spouses, and other sexual partners who might not otherwise be at risk. Probably the only possible positive aspect to the issue of HIV in prison is the fact that within the prison premises, the inmates are a captive audience who may otherwise be hard to reach and may ordinarily avoid seeking health services especially related to HIV due to stigma, fear, criminal policy, etc. As a result, prisons present an opportunity for HIV prevention. Thus, it is essential to address the issue of HIV in prison (Burris & Villena 2004).

Although various efforts have been initiated around the world to tackle the situation of HIV in prisons, the initiatives have remained inadequate. Particularly in India, minimal efforts have been made to deal with the issue of HIV in prison. On one hand, there is a dearth of data and literature on HIV in prisons in the Indian context; on the other hand, the kind of intervention made has remained piecemeal and segregated.

© The Author(s) 2015
S. Guin, *Prison Inmates Living with HIV in India*,
SpringerBriefs in Criminology, DOI 10.1007/978-3-319-15566-1_2

In order to carry out a study on the topic of HIV in prisons, it is imperative to develop an overall understanding about HIV and an insight into the issue of HIV and AIDS in the prisons at national as well as global context. In this chapter, an effort has been made to present the concepts and issues in a comprehensive manner through various subsections capturing all the aspects associated with HIV in prisons, viz. clinical manifestation of HIV and its symptoms, epidemiology of HIV in prisons and preventive measures, vulnerability of prison population to HIV, human rights approach to HIV, and ethical issues regarding HIV in prisons.

Clinical Manifestation of HIV and Its Symptoms

The HIV is a virus that attacks the immune system of the human body. Once the virus infects the human body, the immune system of the person becomes weak, making the body 'immune deficient'. Thus, the immune system becomes incapable of functioning properly and cannot fight other infections, making the body vulnerable to many diseases.

HIV attacks the CD4 cells, a type of white blood cells which are responsible for coordinating the immune system of the body. HIV gradually kills the infected host CD4 cells leading to the production of antibodies. Antibodies are cellular defence mechanism of the human body which fights against unwanted organisms attacking the body. The presence of this antibody in the bloodstream confirms the presence of HIV in a person's body. However, it takes 3 months for the body to produce these antibodies after contracting HIV infection. This 3-month period is called the window period and any HIV test conducted during this window period is negative. Moreover, between 6 days and 6 weeks of HIV infection, the body develops symptoms of other illnesses like fever, enlarged glands, sore throat, aching muscles, and sometimes rashes. These symptoms subside within 2–3 weeks and the person may remain free from these symptoms for over 7–11 years. However, in many cases, these initial symptoms may not occur at all. During these 7–11 years, a person may lead a healthy life without any illnesses. However, the person is now living with HIV and can transmit the virus to other individuals. Over a period of time, usually after 11 years, the virus migrates from the blood circulatory system into the lymph nodes, thrives in the lymph nodes, and continues to infect other CD4 cells. CD4 cells continue to decline on an average of 5–10 % (40–80 cells/cubic mm) per year throughout this phase (Dickson 2001). When the CD4 count of the person living with HIV drops below 200 cells/cubic mm of blood, the body's immune system is completely destroyed. The person is now vulnerable to a large number of infections sometimes called opportunistic infections such as TB, cancer, tumour, etc. In addition to these opportunistic infections, the person may also have fever, weight loss, fatigue, lesions, nausea, and diarrhoea. In most cases, once the CD4 count of the patient drops below 10 cells per cubic millimetre of blood, death ensues (WHO, UNODC, UNAIDS 2008; Dickson 2001; Richards 1999; Cusack & Singh 1994; Thomas 1994).

Origin of HIV

There are several opinions regarding the origin of HIV. According to one opinion, the virus was already present in human body and gradually over a period of time became extremely harmful gradually (Mehta & Sodhi 2004). Others believe it originated from monkeys, chimpanzees, germ warfare laboratory and from a small ethnic group of people (Zeichner & Read 2006).

History of HIV

The existence of AIDS was discovered in October 1980–May 1981 by the Centre for Disease Control in the USA (Jaiswal 1992). HIV was identified in 1983 as the infectious agent responsible for many of the symptoms with illnesses associated with AIDS (Cusack & Singh 1994).

In India, HIV was first recorded in April 1986 among ten female prostitutes from Madras[1] in Tamil Nadu. This was followed by the first AIDS patient in the final stage in May 1986 in Bombay,[2] Maharashtra. This patient was a recipient of unscreened blood transfusion during cardiac surgery in the USA (Kakar 1994; Pavri 1992).

Ways of Transmission of HIV

There are three basic modes of HIV transmission (Dickson 2001; Richards 1999):

1. Unprotected sexual contact: HIV can be transmitted through unprotected sexual intercourse with multiple partners and also through homosexual intercourse between men, if either of the partners is infected. A person having sexually transmitted infection (STI) and engaging in unprotected sexual intercourse may get infected with HIV through open genital sores allowing the virus to enter the bloodstream.
2. Exposure to Infected Blood: Use of non-sterile needle for injecting purposes can cause HIV transmission. HIV is also transmitted through sharing of infected blood and blood products like plasma, red blood cells, etc.
3. Mother to Child Transmission: HIV may also be transmitted from mother to child in womb during pregnancy, during childbirth through exposure to infected maternal blood, and through breastfeeding.

---

[1] Renamed in 1996 to Chennai, the capital city of the Indian state of Tamil Nadu, located in the south of India.
[2] Renamed Mumbai in 1995, the capital city of the Indian state of Maharashtra, located on the west coast of India.

Diagnosis of HIV

Diagnosis of HIV is done through tests that detect the presence of antibodies that a body produces in response to the HIV infection. Two tests, viz. ELISA (Enzyme Linked Immunosorbent Assay) and the Western Blot test, are widely used (Dickson 2001; Richards 1999).

Treatment of HIV

To date there is no specific cure for AIDS. However, usually when the CD4 count drops below 350 cells per cubic millimetre of blood, therapy known as Antiretroviral Therapy (ART) consisting of antiretroviral (ARV) drugs or a combination of three or more antiretroviral drugs, known as Highly Active Antiretroviral Therapy (HAART), is available to increase the CD4 count. These drugs have to be taken everyday for the rest of the life. In the absence of ART or HAART, treatment for opportunistic infections is prescribed, which does not address the immune deficiency (Mehta & Sodhi 2004; Jaiswal 1992).

Prevalence of HIV: Global Scenario

People living with HIV were reported to be 35.3 million worldwide in 2012. There were 2.3 million new HIV infections globally, showing a 33 % decline in the number of new infections from 3.4 million in 2001. The number of AIDS deaths also declined with 1.6 million AIDS deaths in 2012, down from 2.3 million in 2005 (UNAIDS 2013).

Prevalence of HIV: Indian Scenario

It is estimated that in 2011, there were around 20.9 lakh persons living with HIV. Adult HIV prevalence decreased from 0.41 % in 2001 through 0.35 % in 2006 to 0.27 % in 2011. Similarly, the estimated number of people living with HIV decreased from 23.2 lakh in 2006 to 20.9 lakh in 2011. The four high prevalence states of South India (Andhra Pradesh, Karnataka, Maharashtra, and Tamil Nadu) account for 53 % of all persons living with HIV in India (National AIDS Control Organisation 2013).

Prevalence of HIV in Prisons: Global Scenario

Jurgens (2007) documented the prevalence of HIV in prisons in various regions of the world:

> In Eastern Europe and Central Asia, a review of injecting drug users and HIV infection in prisons found HIV prevalence data for all countries, with the exception of Bosnia, Croatia, Turkmenistan, and Uzbekistan (p. 16).

> Lower HIV prevalence was found in prisons in Central Europe, such as in Poland, Czech Republic, Hungary, and Bulgaria, and a much higher prevalence in some of the states of the former Soviet Union—in particular the Russian Federation and Ukraine, but also Lithuania, Latvia, and Estonia. HIV is a growing problem in prisons in some of the states of Central Asia. In South and South East Asia, high prevalence rates are being experienced in some of the countries of this region like Islamic Republic of Iran, Indonesia, Vietnam, and Malaysia, while evidence from India, Pakistan, and Thailand also suggests high rates of HIV among prisoners. The Philippines was the only country for which a study reporting zero prevalence was reported (p. 17).

> In East Asia and the Pacific, overall, little research was done and most of the data available were from China and that too between 8 to 10 years old. In Latin America, HIV prevalence among prisoners in Brazil and Argentina was reported to be particularly high. Rates reported from studies in Mexico, Honduras, Nicaragua, and Panama were also high, although generally lower than in Brazil and Argentina. In the Caribbean, only a small amount of information about HIV prevalence in prisons was available. However, rates reported from Cuba, Jamaica, and Trinidad & Tobago ranged from 4.9 to 25.8 %, suggesting that prevalence among prisoners in this region might be high. In Sub-Saharan Africa, very high prevalence rates were reported from countries in southern Africa, such as Zambia and South Africa and in several western African countries such as Cote d'Ivoire, Gabon, Burkina Faso, Nigeria, and Cameroon. However, in other countries, such as Madagascar, Somalia, Senegal, Mauritius, and Niger, low prevalence was found (p. 18).

> Much of the information on prevalence was more than 5 years old, so it was possible that it did not accurately reflect the current situation of HIV prevalence in African prisons. In North Africa and the Middle East, one study in Yemen in 1998 found an HIV prevalence rate of 26.5 % among a relatively small sample of prisoners. Most other countries for which data were found recorded prevalence of less than one percent. Very little is known about the situation of injecting drug use and HIV among IDUs in prisons in this region. Extensive data exist from many studies undertaken in Western Europe, Australia, Canada, and the USA (p. 19).

Shalihu et al. (2014) observed that most published scientific literature from North America highlights HIV among prisoners. Dolan et al. (2007) reviewed information on HIV prevalence in 152 low-income and middle-income countries in which information on HIV prevalence in prisons was found for 75 countries. Prevalence was greater than 10 % in prisons in 20 countries. Prevalence of IDUs in prison was greater than 10 % in eight countries. HIV prevalence among IDU prisoners was reported in eight countries and was greater than 10 % in seven of those. Evidence of HIV transmission in prison was found for seven low-income and middle-income countries.

Thus, it is evident from the above that HIV infection is a serious problem in prisons throughout the world and should be urgently addressed.

Prevalence of HIV in Prisons: Indian Scenario

Very little data is available regarding the prevalence of HIV in Indian prisons. A case study conducted at the *Mysore jail* in Karnataka—a state with one of the highest prevalence in India—found that the seroprevalence rate was highest among female inmates, at 9.5 %, and 25 % amongst female inmates who were commercial sex workers (Nagaraj et al. 2000 as cited in Goyer 2003). A study of 377 prisoners housed in three prisons in India found that 6.9 % were living with HIV and all of these inmates were originally from Thailand and Myanmar (Pal et al. 1999 as cited in Lines & Stover 2005). Although exact estimates on prevalence of HIV amongst prisoners are not available, 'a bag of the envelope calculation' will suggest that what is commonly present outside the portals of the prison walls should be present inside (Somasundaram & Sundar 1997).

The review of literature by Dolan et al. (2004) revealed that only one study in India found no Injecting Drug Users (IDUs) in one prison, while another found about three inmates (1.2 %) reporting a history of injecting drug use ($n = 249$). Another Indian study found 4.9 % of inmates were IDUs in 1997 and this declined to 0.8 % in 2000. In 1993, 488 IDUs in India who had recently been institutionalized for drug use were tested. The largest centre was Manipur Central Jail, and of those tested, 80 % were HIV positive (UNODC 2007; Dolan et al. 2007).

Dolan & Larney (2010) reviewed various studies (Stubblefield & Wohl 2000; Aggarwal et al. 2005; Sundar et al. 1995; Singh et al. 1999; Nag et al. 2006; Pal et al. 1999; Palaniappan 1995) regarding HIV in prisons in India and noted that existing data for HIV prevalence in prisons were from mid to late 1990s. HIV prevalence in individual prisons ranged from 0.5 to 6.9 %. No information on HIV transmission in Indian prisons was found (Table 2.1). One national study (Nagaraj et al. 2000) of HIV prevalence in prisons found that 1.7 % of male and 9.5 % of female inmates were HIV positive.

From the above, it may be said that data on the prevalence of HIV in Indian prisons are limited. However, the data from the National Crime Records Bureau (2012) clearly show that there is overcrowding in the prisons in India. It must be noted that although the NACO considers Female Sex Workers, Men having Sex with Men, Eunuch/Transgenders, Injecting Drug Users, Long Distance Truckers, and male migrants as high-risk groups, it didn't include prison inmates as one of the high-risk population for the HIV Sentinel Surveillance Round 2008 (National AIDS Control Organisation 2008; International Institute of Population Sciences (IIPS) and Macro International 2007). Thus, in a situation of overcrowding and ignorance regarding HIV among the general population, it is quite apparent that HIV may be quite prevalent in various prisons in India.

Strategies for Preventing HIV in Prisons: Global Scenario

Jurgens (2007) mentioned the following pilot HIV prevention (harm reduction) programmes that were introduced in prisons in many countries throughout the world:

Table 2.1 Information on HIV prevalence in Indian prisons

Location	Year	Sample Size	HIV Prevalence (percent)
Nationally	2000	Unknown	1.7 (total) 9.5 (females)
Amritsar Central Jail	2003	500	2.4
Central Prison, Bangalore	1993	1,114	1.8 (males)
Ghaziabad	1999	249	1.3 (inmates aged 15–50 years)
West Bengal	2000	384	2.3
Orissa, 3 prisons	1994–1995	377	6.9
Chennai	1995	Unknown	3.5
Madurai	1994–1995	Unknown	4.3 (total) 2 (male) 14.2 (female)
Tirunelveli	1995	Unknown	0.5

Source: Dolan & Larney (2010, p. 698)

(a) Mandatory Testing and Segregation: Prisons in the USA, Moldova, Hungary, the Nizhnii Novgorod region of Russia, and Mexico introduced mandatory testing and segregation of known HIV-positive prisoners.

(b) Education: Knowledge about routes of HIV transmission and risks associated with illicit drugs is delivered through prison staffs and prisoners themselves who act as peer educators (UNAIDS 2004)

(c) Condoms: Distribution of condoms to prisoners is permitted in Australia, Brazil, Canada, Ukraine, Moldova, Estonia, Turkmenistan, Romania, and other regions in the Russian Federation, South Africa, very few US prisons (4 city and 2 state systems), and the UK (only via prescription).

(d) Bleach: In order to sterilize injecting equipments, bleach is made available to prisoners in many prisons in Europe.

(e) Needle Exchange or Distribution: Penal Institutions in Western Europe, Central Asia, Switzerland, Germany, Spain, Moldova, Kyrgyzstan, and Belarus distributed syringes via doctors, vending machines, drug counselling services, correctional staff, or external staff.

(f) Tattooing: Guidelines on education and training of prisoner tattoo artist, providing safer tattoo services through a prisoner staffed tattoo shop, and encouraging voluntary screening for blood-borne infectious diseases for tattoo artists have been drafted by the Canadian federal prison system.

(g) Methadone Maintenance Treatment (MMT): Methadone is a long-acting synthetic opiate that is easily absorbed when taken orally once daily. It blocks the effects of the withdrawal symptoms of opium. Thus, MMT discourages the use of non-sterile needle and syringe.

(h) Sexual Health Intervention Strategies: Sexual Health Intervention Strategies were carried out in prisons of Schitomir, Kiev, and Odessa, Ukraine, by conducting training sessions, dissemination of information and educational materials, providing staff and inmates with individual means of protection (disinfectants, condoms, special gloves for staff), establishing regular access to

high-quality STD treatment and counselling, and improving access to psychological assistance and counselling.

(i) HIV and AIDS hotline: In New York, in addition to basic information on transmission and prevention of HIV, regular prevention group meetings, led by a health
educator, were organized. An HIV/AIDS hotline was made available to New York
state prisoners who used a toll-free telephone service designed to be culturally
sensitive. English- and Spanish-speaking counsellors, mostly former prisoners,
gave general information, information about prevention, treatment, and referrals.

Strategies for Preventing HIV in Prisons: Indian Scenario

The following select interventions and research studies have been carried out in
some prisons in India by various governmental and non-governmental organizations
for addressing the issue of HIV in Indian prisons:

The Gujarat State AIDS Control Society, a unit of the National AIDS Control
Organisation, initiated a pilot project on behaviour change communication interventions in 1998 in the Surat District Prison. In 2001, the interventions were replicated
in nine prisons of the state (UNODC 2007).

A study by UNODC (2007) revealed that homosexual activity, both coercive and
consensual, was a reality inside prisons. In this regard, the Hindustan Latex Limited
established a technical resource unit to manage targeted interventions under agree-
ment with the Andhra Pradesh State AIDS Control Society. Initially, four prisons
were selected for the intervention programme, which was upscaled to eight after a
rapid assessment of needs. The intervention focused on behaviour change communication sessions, STD care and counselling, peer education, condom distribution,
and a referral system for partner treatment. The process highlighted the need for
systematic needs assessment and phased upscaling, sensitization, and involvement
of key stakeholders like prison officials and inmates, proper advocacy and sensitization activities, and avoidance of initial media attention in order to provide a greater
sense of privacy, security, and freedom to the concerned project implementers
(UNODC 2007).

Partnerships for Sexual Health Prison projects in Andhra Pradesh: The Prison
Department of Andhra Pradesh in collaboration with the Andhra Pradesh State
AIDS Control Society (APSACS) implemented a project from May 2000 to July
2007 on partnerships for sexual health (PSH) in all prisons of Andhra Pradesh. This
project aimed to bring behavioural change among the prison inmates from the sexual health perspective in the context of STDs and HIV. The project activities
included STD Care and Treatment, STD Counselling, Behaviour Change
Communication (BCC) and peer education, and condom promotion[3] (CHRI 2008).

---

[3] Data obtained from the Office of the Additional Inspector General of Prisons, Hyderabad,
August 2007.

Counselling and Testing by Pune AIDS Control Society: Pune AIDS Control Society (PCACS) was involved in counselling and blood testing of prisoners at the Yerwada Central Prison, Pune, from July 1st 2006 twice a week as per the directives by the Maharashtra State AIDS Control Society and permission given by the Pune Municipal Corporation. PCACS was conducting the tests with pre-test and post-test counselling as per the guidelines of the Maharashtra State AIDS Control Society (MSACS). A copy of the reports was handed to the Superintendent of Prison, Yerwada, Deputy Director of Health Services (DDHS), Pune Circle, and MSACS at the end of each month.[4]

Intervention of NGOs in Prisons: The Commonwealth Human Rights Initiative (CHRI) undertook a National Scoping Study of NGOs working for prison reforms across 14 states in India. The study highlighted examples of best practices ranging from grass-roots level to policy framing. A closer look at the work of the various organizations in various prisons in India highlighted the fact that most of the activities were carried out by the faith-based organizations for education or vocational training, and there were few instances where NGOs occasionally conducted some awareness generation activities. There is a dearth of any concrete and sustainable work related to health per se and HIV and AIDS in particular in prisons by NGOs (CHRI 2008).

Sankalp Rehabilitation Trust is a non-governmental organization addressing the problem of drug abuse in the Mumbai Central Prison and Byculla District Prison in Mumbai, Maharashtra. The organization is involved in providing drug treatment services and legal aid to help inmates who were drug abusers prior to incarceration, through individual counselling, group sessions, medical support, legal intervention, family visits, recreational activities, and training to peer educators.[5]

SAPREM (Social Aspiration for Participatory Reforms by Evolved Manpower), an NGO, initiated the PINJRA (Prevention of HIV/AIDS Infection by Joint Relief Action) Project in Kalyan District Prison, Thane, Maharashtra. The various activities carried out by this NGO in the Kalyan District Prison included behaviour change communication, management of sexually transmitted infections, counselling for HIV testing, and training of peer educators. SAPREM in collaboration with the Tata Institute of Social Sciences, Mumbai, organized a one-day sensitization workshop on the need for HIV & AIDS intervention in prisons on May 12, 2007. The need to organize similar workshops in each state to strengthen care and support on HIV & AIDS intervention in prisons and to frame macro-level policy on HIV & AIDS in prisons emerged as the major recommendations of the workshop (SAPREM n.d.).

Intervention by the Government Hospital: The Department of Preventive and Social Medicine of the L.T.M. Medical College & General Hospital, Sion, Mumbai, was implementing a project on inmates living with HIV. The project included

---

[4] Information collected from the AIDS Nodal Officer and Secretary and counsellors of Pune City AIDS Control Society, 2006.

[5] Information collected through informal discussion with an employee of the organization and researchers' experience of a briefing session by the organization inside the Mumbai Central Prison as a part of the national training programme organized by UNODC and TISS.

counselling session for prisoners living with HIV, pre-test counselling of all prisoners, and conducting HIV-related workshops for the prison staff once a month. The workshops included information regarding the disease, mode of transmission, and treatment.[6]

Efforts by the United Nations Office on Drugs and Crime (UNODC): The UNODC Regional Office for South Asia, New Delhi, in collaboration with Tata Institute of Social Sciences, Mumbai, organized a 5-day national training programme to address HIV prevention amongst incarcerated substance users from February 27 to March 3, 2006. The training was aimed at the Senior/Middle Level Officers from Prisons (Superintendents and Jailors), Police (Anti-Narcotic Cell and the Criminal Investigation Department), and Non-Governmental Organizations from eight Western and Southern States of India. The objective of the programme was to equip the participants with knowledge and information pertaining to substance use and HIV & AIDS in prisons, to sensitize the prison officials and NGOs working on HIV & AIDS prevention in prisons towards the problem of substance use and HIV & AIDS in prison settings, and capacity building of prison officers and other service providers for facilitating training and interventions in the field (UNODC 2006).

In response to the training programme, UNODC and Sankalp organized a one-day sensitization programme regarding HIV & AIDS inside the Mumbai Central Prison premises for the prisoners and staff including the prison personnel, prison medical doctor, and paramedical staff. However, the programme was poorly attended with a few prisoners, prison staff, and paramedical officials.[7]

Vulnerability of Prison Inmates to HIV and the Risk Factors

Socio-economic Conditions

Studies indicate that poverty, unemployment, illiteracy, migration, and displacement may lead to social exclusion facilitating risk behaviour before imprisonment. After imprisonment, they may have language barrier and may have limited access to health information regarding HIV. After release, on deportation to their home countries, they may have limited or no access to prevention, treatment, and medical care services (Lines & Stover 2005).

People living in areas characterized by violence, high rates of crime, and substance abuse are also vulnerable to contract HIV. Apart from substandard housing, overcrowding, and unsanitary living conditions, other factors like unemployment, domestic abuse, dysfunctional relationships, and a lack of security or stability make

---

[6] Information gathered from the prison record on March 23, 2006.

[7] As stated by the programme coordinator on March 15, 2006, based on his observation made during the national training programme.

people vulnerable. Uneducated and the illiterate people do not have access to HIV education programmes (Goyer 2003).

Age, race, and gender are also significant predictors of HIV infection rates. The presence of sexually transmitted infections (STIs) increases the risk of HIV transmission (UNAIDS 1999).

Lack of Awareness

Both the prison inmates and prison staff have negligible or no knowledge on the various aspects of STIs, HIV, and AIDS, like modes of transmission and prevention, symptoms and diagnostic tests, treatment, care, and support. As a result, they are ignorant about the high-risk behaviours they indulge in, which may expose them to HIV (Goyer 2003).

Apart from these, the following pre-incarceration behaviour may render one vulnerable to HIV.

High-Risk Behaviour Prior to Incarceration

High-Risk Behaviour prior to incarceration includes unprotected sex with multiple partners, commercial sex work, or sex in exchange of drugs (Goyer 2003).

Special Target Groups and Vulnerability

Inside the prison, the following sections of people are considered as special target groups vulnerable to contract HIV:

(a) Juvenile Prisoners: Juvenile offenders housed with adult offenders may be sexually abused by the older prison inmates.[8]
(b) Prison Staff: Accidental needle stick injuries from hidden syringes, exposure to human blood or body fluids while administering first aid, indulging in sexual

---

[8] In India, the Juvenile Justice (Care and Protection of Children) Amendment Act, 2006, prescribes provisions for reformation of young offenders till 18 years of age (The Gazette of India 2006) and the Bombay Borstal Schools Act, 1929, provides punishment for the offenders within the age group of 18 to 21 years of age. However, boys found to be too incorrigible or unsociable to be kept in the Borstal School are transferred to the Juvenile Section of the Yerwada Prison (The Gazetteers Department, n.d.). According to these laws, young offenders are to be lodged in the Juvenile Justice Institutions and Borstal Schools, respectively. These places protect them from sexual exploitation by the hardened criminals and/or by the prison warders (which may expose them to HIV).

activities with male prison inmates, and lack of awareness regarding HIV make prison staff vulnerable to HIV (Goyer 2003).

(c) Prison Conditions: Prisons are plagued by overcrowding, decaying physical infrastructure, lack of medical care, guard abuse and corruption, and prisoner on prisoner violence. Poor living conditions, poor opportunities for personal hygiene and sanitation, poor ventilation and natural lighting, and insufficient health-care measures make prisoners at risk to contract TB, a most common opportunistic infection.

(d) Inadequate Prison Medical Facilities: Lack or poorly developed prison medical facilities, inadequate staff, and non-appointment of female doctor for female inmates make it difficult for prison inmates to access health care (Guin 2007).

Risk Behaviour During Incarceration in Prisons

The following behaviours by prison inmates make them vulnerable to HIV infection:

(a) Use of non-sterile injecting equipments: Despite the fact that availability and abuse of drugs are illegal in prisons, drug abuse does happen in various prisons across the world (Jurgens 2007; Goyer 2003). Drug policies which emphasize criminalization over rehabilitation lead to an extremely high incarceration rate amongst drug users and addicts (Goyer 2003).

In the Indian context, the injecting drug users within prisons might be negligible compared to other forms of drug use due to difficulty in smuggling needles and syringes into the prison. However, Singh (2007) notes that anecdotal evidence from previous inmates of the Arthur Road Jail (a jail in Mumbai) had revealed that injecting drug use was common in the jail.

(b) Unprotected sex in prisons: Unprotected sexual activity in prison in the form of consensual (anal intercourse), forced, or coercive (rape) together with the presence of sexually transmitted infections (STIs) makes one vulnerable to contract HIV (Carelse 1994). Sex may also be used as a form of currency exchanged for money, protection, space, property, or drugs within the prison. Other factors like whether the accommodation is single cell or dormitory, the duration of the sentence, the security classification, and the extent to which conjugal visits are permitted also influence sexual activity (Lines & Stover 2005). It has to be noted here that Indian prison does not allow conjugal visits by law.

Since sodomy is illegal in Indian prisons, MSM is not openly discussed due to fear of punishment from the prison authorities and stigmatization. Thus, there are no data available neither on its occurrence nor on its frequency (Lines & Stover 2005; Goyer 2003).

In many societies, homosexuality is not an accepted behaviour and social stigma is attached to this sexual orientation. As a result, prisoners engaged in homosexual activities are discriminated by other fellow prisoners and prison staff. This inhibits such prisoners to access safe sex measures such as condoms (in prisons where condom is made available). Moreover, sexual activity in any form (consensual or coercive) is prohibited under the Prison Act of many countries, which is an impediment for inmates to access safer sex practices or seek medical care for any STI or venereal diseases. Existing studies conducted in different countries across the globe (Australia, Sweden, Austria, Spain, Belgium, Britain, the USA, Philadelphia, Malawi, Zomba) have revealed that the prevalence of high-risk sexual behaviour in prisons is quite high (Lines & Stover 2005; Goyer 2003).

(c) Use of Non-sterile equipments (body art/shaving): Though any form of body art by the inmates (tattooing, body piercing, etc.) is illegal, it is an integral part of the prison culture in many countries like Australia, Canada, Ireland, Spain, and the USA. In order to ensure that none of the participants get caught by the prison staff, these activities are usually done in a hurry in secret places (which in a prison are obviously very unhygienic) using non-sterile equipments (Lines & Stover 2005; UNAIDS 2004). Moreover, in undeveloped/developing countries, many prisoners share razors for shaving purposes, which increase the likelihood of exposure to blood-borne diseases (UNAIDS 2004).

(d) Exposure to human blood and body fluids: Prisoner and prison staff may get exposed to HIV-infected blood and body fluids through assaults, fights, accidental needle stick injuries or concealed syringes, and while providing first aid (Lines & Stover 2005):

The above high-risk behaviours inside the prison may be major causes of HIV transmission in prisons.

HIV-Related Diseases

(a) TB Infection: TB is the most common opportunistic infection for prisoners living with HIV (World Health Organization 2014; Dara et al. 2009; UNAIDS 2004).

India has one of the largest TB population in the world and prisons in India report TB as a major health problem. Many inmates contract the disease after entering the prison. With already weakened immune systems, inmates living with HIV are vulnerable to any infection. TB infection poses a great threat to the general health of inmates living with HIV. Thus, housing these inmates along with those with TB greatly heightens the risk of contracting TB. The risk of the spread of TB is also heightened by poorly ventilated and overcrowded prison conditions. Thus, high rates of HIV and other infectious diseases like TB can lead to alarmingly high rates of mortality among prisoners.

(b) Hepatitis B/Hepatitis C (HCV) Infection: Hepatitis B and C are two forms of Hepatitis. These are transmitted through the use of non-sterile syringes and other injection equipments. Hepatitis B can also be transmitted through unprotected sexual activity or in any situation where blood or body fluids from an infected person enter the body of a person who is not immune. A vaccine is available to prevent Hepatitis B, but there is no vaccine to prevent Hepatitis C (Macalino et al. 2004).

Published studies of HCV in the prison setting include those from Australia, Taiwan Province of China, India, Ireland, Denmark, Scotland, Greece, Spain,

England, Brazil, the USA, and Canada. Majority of these studies have reported that 20–40 % of prisoners were living with HCV, and within study samples, rates of HCV prevalence among prisoners who were injecting drug users were usually two to three times higher than those who have no history of injecting drug use (Macalino et al. 2004).

(c) Sexually Transmitted Infections (STIs): Inmates suffering from STIs are at higher risk of contracting HIV infection and people living with HIV are more susceptible to STI, due to their weak immune system (Lines & Stover 2005; UNAIDS 2004).

Prohibitory Law and Availability of Resources

In countries and prison systems where homosexuality is legal, like Australia, Brazil, Canada, Indonesia, the Islamic Republic of Iran, South Africa, some countries of the former Soviet Union, and a few prison systems in the USA, prison inmates have access to condoms (Jurgens 2007).

In India, homosexuality is a punishable offence under Section 377 of the Indian Penal Code. Naz Foundation, an NGO fighting for the gay rights in India, challenged the validity of Section 377, India's anti-sodomy law, before a division bench of Chief Justice A.P. Shah and Justice Murlidharan of the Delhi High Court.[9] In response to the petition by The Naz Foundation (India) Trust, the Delhi High Court had decriminalized adult consensual sexual acts in private in 2009. However, the Supreme Court in Suresh Kumar Koushal v. Naz Foundation upheld the validity of Section 377, IPC, in December, 2013. The Naz Foundation (India) Trust filed a curative petition challenging the Supreme Court judgement (Naz Foundation files Curative Petition 2014).

Possession of addictive drugs is an offence in India under the Narcotic Drugs and Psychotropic Substances Act 1985 (NDPS). Thus, the two of the major modes of transmission of HIV in prisons, homosexuality and injecting drug use, are illegal in India. As a result, provision of resources for STD/HIV/AIDS prevention such as condoms, water-based lubricants, sterile syringes, needles, bleach, or other disinfectants for cleaning the injecting equipment cannot be distributed within the prison (Singh 2007).

Lack of Confidentiality

Confidentiality of medical information during imprisonment is difficult to maintain and is often breached, especially if it concerns STD/HIV/AIDS. In this study, it was observed that in some prisons, confidentiality regarding HIV-positive status could

---

[9]Naz Foundation (India) Trust v. Government of NCT, Delhi and Others [Writ Petition (Government) No. 7455 of 2001].

not be maintained mainly due to the special diet that inmates were provided with. In one prison, 'HIV positive' was marked on the medical files of the HIV-positive inmates. Apart from the doctor, HIV-positive inmates were identifiable by the nursing staff in the prison and the police guards who escorted the prisoners to the Government hospitals when referred. Medical personnel were not trained regarding the importance of privacy and confidentiality.[10] Thus, there is very little understanding about the fact that prison inmates have greater need for privacy because they live in closed community where stigmatization, suicide, and violence are common.

Lack of Policy Guidelines on HIV in Prisons

In India, each State has its own prison manual based on the Model Prison Manual of 1960, which obviously was formulated long before HIV was discovered. As a result, each of these State prison manuals lacks any guidelines to address HIV in prisons. The only mention of HIV/AIDS in any policy document relating to the prison administration in India is in the Model Prison Manual 2003 and the National Policy on Prison Reforms and Correctional Administration, framed by the Bureau of Police Research and Development (BPR&D). It suggests provision of isolation rooms to house inmates suffering from contagious diseases like TB, Leprosy, and HIV/AIDS, in each prison hospital (Bureau of Police Research and Development 2003). This guideline, in fact, is more detrimental for an inmate living with HIV who is free from any other co-infection, as it exposes him/her to all other contagious diseases. Moreover, there is no mention of HIV/AIDS in prison setting in the draft report on the National Policy on Criminal Justice framed by the Ministry of Home Affairs (Government of India 2007).

Interestingly, the National AIDS Control Organisation, set up by the Government of India under the Ministry of Health and Family Welfare, in 1992, to address each and every aspect of HIV and AIDS in the country, including ethical aspects, prevention, treatment, care, and support, has completely ignored the incidence of HIV within prisons (National AIDS Control Organisation 2013).

Human Rights Perspective

There are three broad areas which highlight the relationship between HIV and human rights (OHCHR 1996–2004).

(a) Increased vulnerability: The vulnerability of certain groups of people increases if they are unable to exercise their political, economic, social, and cultural

---

[10] Observation of the researcher during data collection in December 2006 for M.Phil. research study on, 'HIV/AIDS in Prisons: A Human Rights Perspective'.

rights. For example, if the Right to Information is denied to people, they will not be able to access information related to HIV.

(b) Discrimination and stigma: Discrimination and stigma related to HIV may deny rights to people living with HIV. Stigmatization and discrimination may not only obstruct their access to treatment but may also affect their employment, housing, and other rights.

(c) Impedes an effective response: If human rights of vulnerable groups such as injecting drug users, sex workers, and men who have sex with men are not respected, strategies to combat HIV & AIDS epidemic will never yield the expected outcome.

International Mechanisms

The provisions under international mechanisms ensure all the rights of prisoners except the ones they must be deprived of under legal provisions, for the sake of incarceration. There are two general categories of instruments that protect human rights. Each poses different obligations on governments. International human rights law and International rules, standards, and guidelines are the two international instruments that protect the human rights of all groups of people globally, the former being binding on governments (Betteridge 2004).

International Human Rights Laws

The States which ratify these international human rights laws are legally bound to frame laws that ensure respect, protection, and fulfilment of the right of prisoners (life, equality, security, privacy, etc.) and legal provisions for effective measures in case of violation of rights (in case of cruel, inhuman, or degrading treatment) (Betteridge 2004).

International Rules, Standards, and Guidelines

The most important rules, standards, and guidelines in relation to prison inmates are as follows (Betteridge 2004):

1. Basic Principles for the Treatment of Prisoners
2. Body of Principles for the Protection of All Persons under Any Form of Detention or Imprisonment

3. Standard Minimum Rules for the Treatment of Prisoners
4. Recommendation No R (98) 7 of the Committee of Ministers to Member States Concerning the Ethical and Organisational Aspects of Health Care in Prison

The other international instruments in the context of HIV & AIDS in prisons are as follows:

1. The World Health Organization (WHO) Guidelines on HIV Infection and AIDS in Prisons, 1993: In 1987, the WHO came up with its first recommendation to address HIV in prison. In 1993, WHO published another guideline which focused on voluntary testing, confidentiality, non-discrimination of HIV-positive inmates, availability of the means of prevention, and access to treatment equivalent to that in the community (UNAIDS 1999).

2. International Guidelines on HIV/AIDS, 1996: The Guideline 4 of the International Guidelines on HIV/AIDS and Human Rights has a section which emphasizes the administrative measures the prison authorities must take to ensure protection of inmates from rape, sexual violence, and coercion. It also recommended provision of information and education on HIV prevention, voluntary testing, and means of prevention (condoms, bleach, and sterile injection equipment), treatment, and care not only to inmates but to prison staff as well. It suggested prohibition of mandatory testing, solitary confinement, and restricting the access to prison facilities. The guidelines included provision for voluntary participation of inmates in clinical trials on HIV and early release of HIV-positive inmates on compassionate grounds (UNAIDS 2006).

3. United Nations General Assembly Special Session on HIV/AIDS (UNGASS), June 2001: The UNGASS Declaration of Commitment identified four areas: prevention of new infections, provision of improved care, support, and treatment for those infected with and affected by HIV/AIDS, reduction of vulnerability, and mitigation of the social and economic impact of HIV/AIDS to reverse the epidemic by 2015. Strengthening of monitoring mechanisms for HIV/AIDS-related human rights violations was acknowledged (UNAIDS 2002).

4. The Dublin Declaration on HIV/AIDS in Prisons in Europe and Central Asia, 2004: With a broader focus to ensure the rights of prisoners to HIV prevention and treatment, the Irish Penal Reform Trust in collaboration with experts from seven different countries proposed guidelines to deal with HIV in prisons based on best practices to address the issue, scientific evidence, and a human rights perspective. Over 90 NGOs and experts in the field of Criminology and HIV and AIDS endorsed the declaration (The Dublin Declaration on HIV/AIDS in Prisons in Europe and Central Asia 2005).

5. Global Fund to Fight AIDS, Tuberculosis, and Malaria: The present focus of global efforts to address HIV and AIDS is universal access to comprehensive prevention programmes, treatment, care, and support. Many countries committed themselves towards this end in the 2005 World Summit and 2006 High Level Meeting on AIDS. Global Fund to Fight AIDS, Tuberculosis, and Malaria is one of the major initiatives to ensure funds for extensive response.

National Mechanisms

National AIDS Control Programme

Since the inception of NACP Phase-I (NACP-I), based on the changing trends of the HIV epidemic in India, NACO has been shifting the focus of the National AIDS Control Programme (NACP) in each of its subsequent phases (NACP II, NACP III, etc.). Presently behaviour change has replaced awareness generation. With active engagement and participation of NGOs and Positive (HIV positive) Networks (PLHIV) across the country, NACP has turned into a more decentralized response. NACP-IV, launched in April 2012, aims to accelerate the process of reversal and to further strengthen the epidemic response in India through a cautious and well-defined integration process over 5 years 2012–2017 (National AIDS Control Organisation 2013).

The HIV/AIDS Bill 2007

The Lawyers Collective HIV/AIDS Unit drafted the HIV/AIDS Bill 2007. The Bill proposes provision of and access to risk reduction strategies, counselling, and health-care services for prisoners and detainees services (Lawyers Collective HIV/AIDS Unit 2008).

HIV Jurisprudence in India

A few of the landmark judgements given by the Indian Judiciary in cases involving people living with HIV are (Krishnan 2003):

- In 1990 the Bombay High Court ruled in favour of isolation of AIDS patient, but made it mandatory to ensure the hearing of a person living with HIV who has been detained.
- A very significant public policy ruling was given by the Supreme Court of India in 1996, through which an order was issued for all the state governments, the central government, and NACO to bring about a series of changes.
- The judgement against the discrimination at workplace of the people living with HIV was given by the Bombay High court in 1997 that an employer cannot consider an applicant or an existing employee unfit for the job/position unless the HIV status of the person interferes with her/his job performance.
- The Assam High Court ordered the government agencies working on HIV/AIDS to have more transparency and accountability in their work/programmes.

- The High Court in Kerala directed NACO to release its work and findings on AIDS to the public.
- The Calcutta High Court issued an interim order directing the Indian Navy to pay compensation to a family where the wife of a Naval officer contracted HIV during her blood transfusion in a military hospital.
- In 1998, Sahara House, a centre for Residential Care and Rehabilitation and in 1999 Sankalp Rehabilitation Trust (through Lawyers Collective), filed two separate but similar PILs in the Supreme Court, to ensure that no person living with HIV or is suspected to be HIV positive was denied treatment in the Government-run hospitals. On 1st October, 2008, the Hon'ble Supreme Court passed interim directions and directed the State Governments and NACO to implement the interim directions in a timely fashion (Sahara House vs. Union of India, [W.P, (C) No. 535 of 1998]; Sankalp Rehabilitation Trust vs. Union of India, [W.P. (C) No. 512 of 1999].

Initiatives Taken by the National Human Rights Commission

The National Human Rights Commission (NHRC) has taken up various initiatives to protect the Human Rights of people living with HIV/AIDS. NHRC secured proper medical treatment to an AIDS patient at a Government Hospital in Delhi and directed that in medical cases dealing with HIV-positive patients, hospitals should offer proper treatment to the poor patients.

The Commission in partnership with other key agencies (National AIDS Control Organisation, the Lawyers Collective, the UN Children's Fund, and the UN Joint Programme) organized the National Conference on Human Rights and HIV/AIDS in New Delhi in November 2000. The recommendations emerging from the conference were formulated as *action points*. Some of these action points were on consent and testing of HIV, confidentiality, discrimination in health care and employment, women in vulnerable environments, children and young people, people living with HIV/AIDS (PLHA), marginalized populations, etc. These action points respond to the issue of HIV/AIDS both on national and state levels, in reference to all partners, including the international and domestic non-governmental organizations, foreign governments and multilateral agencies, credit institutions, the business community/private sector, employers' and workers' associations, religious associations, and communities. Another purpose of the *action points* is to complement the International Guidelines on HIV/AIDS and Human Rights with practical solutions in the Indian context. Based on the deliberations of the National Conference, systemic recommendations on various aspects of 'Human Rights and HIV/AIDS' were sent to the concerned authorities in the Central Government, State Governments, NGOs, and other key stakeholders (National Human Rights Commission 2006).

The Commission mounted a multimedia campaign to disseminate information on the Human Rights and HIV/AIDS to various target groups. In this direction, the Commission published 'Know Your Rights' series on Human Rights and HIV/

AIDS in collaboration with the National Academy of Legal Studies and Research University (NALSAR), Hyderabad, and produced a short duration film entitled 'HIV/AIDS—Myth and Reality' from a Human Rights perspective in partnership with Doordarshan (National Human Rights Commission 2006).

HIV in Prisons: Ethical Issues

While conducting research involving prison inmates living with HIV, the following ethical issues must be taken into consideration (Williams 2008):

1. Informed Consent and Voluntary Testing: Any person who is tested for HIV should be given complete information about the nature of the test and its implications. A policy on voluntary testing has been framed by NACO, which mandates pre- and post-test counselling (National AIDS Control Organisation 2008).
2. Informed Consent for Research: Any research which involves people living with HIV should ensure that all the participants are fully informed about all the various aspects of the research (purpose, funding, organization/institution involved, duties and responsibilities of the researcher, method of record keeping, absence of any physical incentive, risks, benefits, etc.) and their consent (based on the information) is taken, before the research is conducted, with a guarantee of confidentiality of each of the participants.
3. Confidentiality vs. Disclosure: On one hand, it is the right of the prison inmate living with HIV that his/her HIV status is kept confidential, and on the other hand, it is the moral and legal responsibility of the State, including the prison administration, to ensure that the prison staff, other inmates, and the community (where the inmate will go back after release) are protected from getting infected with HIV. Hence, the priority that should be given to keep the inmate's HIV status confidential in order to protect him/her from threat, stigma, and discrimination is no less than the priority that should be given to ensure preventive measures for others and treatment measures for the inmate living with HIV. Presently, there is no clear directive of the Prison Administration regarding the process that should be followed to ensure both these aspects.
4. Segregation and Mainstreaming: There are two aspects favouring segregation—the inmates living with HIV are more prone to other infections compared to the other inmates and it has been observed that some inmates living with HIV engage in reckless behaviour in a deliberate attempt to infect others. On the other hand, a blanket segregation of all inmates living with HIV will lead to exclusion, which will only increase the distress of the already suffering inmate. However, it would be better if the segregation of the prisoner is based on the assessment of each individual cases, considering the medical status, need for protection, and likelihood of engaging in reckless behaviours (Somasundaram & Sundar 1997).

Conclusion

It is evident from the above that there are a good many number of factors which make the study of prison inmates living with HIV not only conclusively significant but also a prerequisite to ensure that the policies and legal provisions are introduced for safeguarding the interests of these inmates in prisons in particular and the community in general. HIV is a very serious and delicate issue inside the prison because of the risk behaviours prison inmates engage in during their term inside the prison as well as after their release to the community. Both prison inmates as well as the prison staff are vulnerable to HIV inside the prison. Although there exist a considerable number of institutional mechanisms in relation to HIV in general and HIV in prisons in particular, the implementation of these mechanisms in the domestic scenario is a matter of investigation. In India, the National AIDS Control Organisation is the only body of the Government of India to address issues relating to HIV and AIDS. Although the HIV/AIDS Bill is the only legislation that has been initiated, there is no particular policy or legislation with regard to HIV in prisons. In this context, it is important to find out the various issues and facets related to HIV and AIDS in prisons giving special emphasis on prisoners' access to healthy conditions, prevention, and treatment.

Chapter 3
Profile of Prison Inmates Living with HIV

Before proceeding to analyse the experiences of prison inmates living with HIV, it is essential to understand the background of these prison inmates. As evident from the literature review, research on the situation of prison inmates living with HIV has been very limited in the Indian context. As a result, there is a paucity of empirical data and literature on prison inmates living with HIV, in India.

The present research uses case study research method. Yin (2009) defines the case study research method as 'an empirical inquiry about a contemporary phenomenon (e.g. a "case"), set within its real-world context—especially when the boundaries between phenomenon and context are not clearly evident'.

This chapter presents the seven case studies developed on the basis of the data collected through qualitative interview. The interview data have been transformed into narratives. The case narratives have been presented in the form of case studies. These case studies will vividly provide a detailed account of the background of the prison inmates living with HIV, within the scope of the study.

Case Study I: Raja[1]

Raja, 35 years old, hailed from Thane[2] district of Maharashtra. Before being imprisoned, he used to live with his mother, brother, and sister. His father, who used to work in the railways, had passed away. After his incarceration, his mother stayed with his brother in Mumbai and the married sister lived with her in-laws. Raja was a bachelor. He felt that it was good that he never got married as he would have

---

[1] Names have been changed. All study participants chose or were assigned a pseudonym.

[2] Thane is a district situated in the north of Maharashtra, a state in western India.

© The Author(s) 2015
S. Guin, *Prison Inmates Living with HIV in India*,
SpringerBriefs in Criminology, DOI 10.1007/978-3-319-15566-1_3

ruined his wife's life as well, considering the fact that he landed up in prison and had been diagnosed with HIV. Had he been married, his wife would have been in trouble as there would have been no one to look after her.

Raja studied till standard IX in a Marathi[3] medium school, after which he lost interest in his studies. He started working as a salesman, in the year 1985, in a Government-recognized agency. This agency was engaged in checking of various weighing machines. He worked there for 13 years and used to earn around Rs. 2,000 per month.

He was charged in a murder case, along with his friends, and thus landed up in prison. He was convicted on February 3, 2000, and sentenced with rigorous life imprisonment. He was serving the tenth year of his imprisonment at the time of interview.

After being convicted, he was allotted work in the prison hospital. He served there for 3 years. During these 3 years, he was fit and fine. Later, he once suffered from prolonged illness with rashes all over his body. He suspected himself to be HIV infected, as he knew that people who were HIV positive usually developed boils and it was one of the most common symptoms of HIV. He informed the same to the prison doctor and requested him for a blood test to confirm the HIV status. The prison doctor collected his blood sample and sent it to the National AIDS Research Institute (NARI).[4] The test result confirmed that he was HIV positive. His blood was tested a second time at the government hospital, for further confirmation. This report reconfirmed his HIV status. Prior to the test, he was explained by the concerned HIV counsellor regarding the nature of the test. However, initially, the test report was not revealed to him. It was only when he insisted for it that he was disclosed of his HIV-positive status by one of his 'friends', a fellow prisoner working as a nurse at the prison hospital. He was recommended to eat nutritious food and have medicines on time.

Prior to incarceration, Raja had the habit of drinking occasionally. He used to visit brothels and had unprotected sexual contact with many (as many as 20/25) women. At that time, he didn't know about HIV. He had no information about how HIV spreads and the preventive measures that should be taken to minimize its spread. He became aware of the disease when he was serving the seventh year of his term.

Raja was receiving the special diet meant for sick prisoners. At around 6.45 a.m., he was served 400 ml milk (meant for the medical patients, the usual quota being 100 ml milk for other prisoners) and around 7 a.m. he was served tea. At around 9 a.m., his platter included four breads, one sweet lime, two bananas, and one egg. Lunch was served at around 10.30 in the morning which consisted of rice (one bowl), four *chappatis* (handmade wheat bread), cooked *daal* (lentils), and a

---

[3] Marathi is the official language of Maharashtra.

[4] National AIDS Research Institute (NARI) was established in October 1992 in Pune, Maharashtra, India, to achieve prevention and control of HIV and provide care and support to HIV-infected population.

vegetable curry. The same food was served, around 4.30 in the evening, as dinner. He commented that the quality of food served was very poor in terms of the spices (*masala*) used for cooking, as the food was quite hot (spicy). Since he suffered from mouth ulcers, it was difficult for him to eat this spicy food. He felt that the food should be so cooked that the inmates living with HIV could easily consume and digest. He believed that the only treatment, which could be given to a HIV-positive person, was proper food with high-protein content.

Raja lamented that he was neither receiving high-protein diet nor any medication. Although he was aware that there was no cure for the disease, yet he knew that one could stay healthy for a longer period of time with proper diet and medication. For him, receiving proper diet was equivalent to receiving some kind of medical treatment for this incurable disease. He conveyed that many HIV-positive inmates in the prison were receiving medicines and treatment for HIV.

> I am aware that many inmates living with HIV are receiving medicines and protein-rich diet. But I am not getting any. I do not want to get into conflict with anyone as I know that I will not live long. I try to live with a free mind without any kind of unnecessary tension. If I am destined to die a slow and pathetic death due to this incurable disease, then I will have to, as this is the punishment for all my wrong deeds.

Since the last 6 years, he had lumps behind his left ear and some other parts of his body. He wanted to get these operated, but the doctors were not ready to operate on him because of his HIV status. Instead, he was given some medicines for the same. However, as these medicines were ineffective, he said that sometimes he wanted to cut these lumps open with a blade to remove whatever was inside. But he never did it, since he knew that it would not solve the problem.

When Raja was diagnosed with HIV, he had also contracted TB, the most common co-infection. He underwent DOTS[5] treatment for a period of one and half years. Afterwards, his blood sample was sent to the government hospital for TB test, but he never received the report.

> No one was there to follow it up. Sassoon (name of the government hospital) is a busy place with lots of patients. Also, the doctors there behave in a very strange way, as I am a prisoner and more so, as I am HIV positive.

However, during the second session of the interview, 2 months later, Raja confirmed that he was completely cured of TB. He said that there was no problem for inmates suffering from TB and the TB treatment in the prison was the best.

The behaviour of fellow inmates towards Raja did not change despite his HIV status. He shared the following observation regarding access to information on HIV, engagement in work, and the discriminatory practices in the prison.

> All the inmates stayed together and information on HIV reached the prisoners through newspapers, TV and other sources. People, who were HIV positive but were capable of working, were allowed to work in the various workshops and factories inside the prison. However, there were some people who treated them in a discriminatory way. There was a

---

[5] DOTS or Direct Observatory Treatment with Short Course Chemotherapy is the internationally recommended TB control strategy.

general tendency, of ill-treatment of sick and ailing prisoners, by the medical staff. This was irrespective of the patient's HIV status. The doctors examined the patient from a distance and prescribed medicine on a random basis.

The main problem that he faced was the food. There were times when he was unable to eat any food due to mouth ulcers. Moreover, at times, he experienced severe pain in the joints. Even the slightest discomfort in the body troubled him as his mind was always preoccupied thinking about the disease.

Once in a while he came across TV programmes on HIV. There were some posters on HIV, which were on display inside the office of the medical ward. But there was no one to reach out to, with whom he could share and discuss his health condition and problems. He tried to make himself comfortable within the available resources. He expressed that in cases like his, even talking to someone, once in a while, was of great help.

Inside the prison, he felt helpless as he could not access proper treatment on his own. He conveyed that if any community-based group wanted to help him, he was willing to seek their help for medical care, for psychological support, and for facilitating integration in the community. He recalled that sometime back, a video on HIV was screened. He said that if there were people from any NGO who were interested to talk on HIV and AIDS, then, even prisoners who were not infected with HIV would be willing to discuss on the subject. There were no voluntary agencies that visited the prison to spread the awareness on HIV.

> I really wish there were organizations to help people suffering from HIV/AIDS. After my release, I would be eager to get in touch and seek the help of any such organization willing to lend a helping hand. Are you aware of any such organization?

For undergoing continued treatment, allotment of police guard as escorts to the government hospital[6] posed a major hindrance. He shared that the behaviour of doctors was discriminatory and rude.

> …very few inmates (HIV positive) are on medication. Police guards are rarely allotted. OPD closes at 12 p.m. at Sassoon hospital. By the time I reach OPD, its already past 12 p.m. If I can reach before 12, they send me to another department. But the availability of doctor in the various departments is very uncertain. And the doctors talk very rudely. Being educated, if they behave in this manner, what can be expected of others?

Raja was aware of the symptoms, causes, and consequences of HIV. He shared:

> This disease is such that the symptoms start to appear only about 7–8 years after getting infected. Most of the cases are like this. There was an inmate who was HIV positive and survived his whole life term inside the prison without having any problem. He was released after completing his whole term of imprisonment. The disease is such that, sometimes, the patient suffers from very high fever for a prolonged period——a minimum period of one and a half months. Then, there are boils all over the body, one loses the appetite and has to go to the toilet frequently. The disease is transmitted through unprotected sexual contact with multiple partners. The other route of spread, of this disease, is through infected blood.

---

[6] The government hospital in the city/town where the prison is located and where the inmates are referred to for treatment by the prison medical doctor.

He expressed his desire for better treatment.

> I think I should start getting medication for HIV at the earliest. If I was outside the prison, I could have done something to get myself treated. But inside the prison, there is no treatment available for those living with HIV. Last month, I saw in the newspaper that there is a medicine which is available for the disease, but inside the prison nothing is provided, and the food is of such quality that it is very difficult to eat and digest.

Case Study II: Ram[7]

Ram was from Midnapur district of West Bengal. He came to Mumbai when he was 18 and had been living in the city since the last 11 years. His family comprised of his father, mother, and three sisters. He was not married. His father worked as a salesman in a jewellery shop in Kolkata. Two of his sisters were married and stayed with their in-laws, one in Delhi and the other in Punjab. The third one was studying in standard tenth and lived at home. His two uncles stayed in Mumbai and maternal uncle lived in Kolkata.

He had studied till class IV. He was working as a helper in a jewellery shop before being incarcerated. He got hands-on training in jewellery-making at the age of 10. He started working and learning jewellery-making at Boubazar in Kolkata. Someone living in his neighbourhood had a jewellery shop in Mumbai and was looking for a person to work in his shop. Ram's mother went to him and offered to send Ram with him to Mumbai to work in his shop. Since Ram knew the work, the person agreed and Ram accompanied him to Mumbai in 1996. During the first year, he used to earn Rs. 2,500 per month as salary. Moreover, each month he used to procure 1–2 gms of gold through the work. As a result, his total monthly income was around Rs. 7,000. He used to send some money home, used some amount for his own expenditure, and deposited the rest in the bank. He had the habit of occasionally consuming beer and smoking cigarette.

It was during this period that he got into the habit of visiting 'beer dance bars'.[8] He started going to these bars along with his friends and developed sexual relationship with the bar dancers. He was all alone in Mumbai and used to get too disturbed by his family tensions. Afterwards, he started visiting these bars alone, without any influence from anyone else.

He wanted to go to Dubai to earn more money. For this, he gave an advance of Rs. 25,000 to an agent, who was supposed to arrange for the travel and work in Dubai. The agent had asked for a total amount of Rs 30,000 and had promised to arrange everything for him. Ram had also given the agent his ration card, school leaving certificate, and passport photographs. But for 9 months, every time Ram

---

[7] Names have been changed. All study participants chose or were assigned a pseudonym.

[8] A 'bar' is a business establishment that serves alcoholic drinks. Some bars have entertainment on a stage, such as a live band, comedians, or dancers. In many bars, the bar dancers are commercial sex workers.

went to the agent, the agent told that his work will be done and kept on postponing. In the meantime, a Gujarati neighbour of Ram offered him to start a workshop where he could make gold ornaments. The Gujarati neighbour offered to provide him financial remuneration in lieu of his expertise. Ram found this to be a good opportunity to work independently and earn more money. He decided to call off his plans to go to Dubai. He asked the agent to give him the money back so that he could concentrate on this new offer. But the agent refused to return the money. This resulted in a heated argument. In a fit of anger, Ram killed the agent. After the murder, he fled to Kolkata. One of his maternal uncles disclosed his whereabouts to the police and he was arrested from his Midnapur house in West Bengal.

Ram was convicted for life on charges of murder on August 31, 1999, and was brought to the prison on October 9, 1999. He had already undergone imprisonment as an undertrial with effect from May 13, 1996, till August 30, 1999, a period of 3 years 3 months and 19 days, which was counted within the sentence period.

Inside the prison, he used to exercise regularly and was maintaining a good health. It was in 2003 when he started suffering from body ache, fever, and vomiting accompanied with severe weakness and was referred to the government hospital by the then Chief Medical Officer (CMO) for check-up. He was tested for HIV. However, he was not informed anything about the nature and reason for the test, and the test report was not disclosed to him. He came to know that he was HIV positive when he approached one of his friends (fellow prisoner) who used to work in the CMO's office. By this time, he had seen other HIV patients and was aware that it is an incurable disease. As mentioned, he did not receive any pre- or post-test counselling about the preventive and other health measures to be followed in order to live fit, fine, and healthy to the maximum extent possible.

He wanted to keep his HIV status confidential. However, somehow, a few fellow prisoners came to know about his HIV status. When probed about the source of the information, he said that most of the inmates drew the conclusion based on the separate medical diet, meant for the ailing prisoners, that he was receiving. According to him, there were three different kinds of diet that were being given to inmates—one for those living with HIV, one for the diabetic patients, and the third kind was the normal diet meant for those who did not have any medical condition. Hence, the other inmates came to know of his HIV-positive status on the basis of the special diet. He also expressed that when it came to food, some inmates were not happy that Ram was getting a special diet, which they were deprived of. But apart from this issue, other inmates did not have any grudge against him. Mostly, they ignored the fact that he was HIV positive. But sometimes the warders[9] and prison guards did not talk to him properly. However, this had nothing to do with his HIV status. It was a general behaviour of the Chief Medical Officer, the prison warders, and the guards, towards every inmate; they talked rudely with the prisoners.

He didn't tell his family in West Bengal that he was HIV positive because he didn't want to bother his parents. He was regularly in touch with his family through

---

[9] Convicted long-term prisoners are appointed as prison warders based on certain criteria according to Maharashtra Prison Manual, 1979.

letters and very rarely through phone calls, which he managed to make when he was referred to the government hospital for treatment. When the researcher asked if he had seen his medical record file, he informed that his medical record file was kept with the CMO. He was willing to disclose his medical information to the prison staff and judicial authority if such information was used for his benefit—prison transfer to West Bengal prison.

He shared that when he was referred to the government hospital for treatment of tuberculosis, the response of the doctor was very hurtful. According to him, doctors treated prisoners with great hatred irrespective of their HIV status.

He was working as a tailor in the prison tailoring section, for which he was earning a wage at the rate of Rs. 25 for sewing 6 shirts in 7 hours. But he was more interested in designing jewellery and did not like the work of a tailor. 10 % of his wage was deposited in his account in the prison office, which he would receive at the time of release. The rest of the money, which he could keep inside the prison, was in the form of coupons. This coupon could be utilized for buying food in the prison canteen. Ram worked whenever his health permitted. So based on the attendance in the workshop, he had to fill up a form, and depending upon the number of days of work, he received his wage.

There was no restriction on prison inmates living with HIV from accessing any recreational facilities available, like volleyball and carrom board.

He was aware of HIV and AIDS and knew how the disease spreads. He got informed about HIV and AIDS during his stay in the prison through other inmates living with HIV, and from TV and newspapers. He had a habit of collecting newspaper cuttings on HIV and AIDS. He was never told about any treatment options. The Medical Officer decided the course of treatment for every ailing inmate. Ram had seen few posters in the hospital ward on HIV and AIDS. But apart from this, there was no other information available inside the prison. There were some 'good' people among the inmates whom he had befriended. One such friend had informed him about an Ayurvedic[10] treatment for HIV and AIDS, which was available in Kerala. His friend had promised that he would help Ram in procuring the medicine from Kerala. When asked, whether this friend of his would charge any money for this favour, Ram said that he wouldn't as they were friends.

Ram had tuberculosis and skin disease. He was cured of TB after undergoing DOTS treatment.

Ram had never received any medication for HIV. Getting a guard, as escort to the government hospital, was always difficult.

Ram received food thrice a day. At around 6.30 in the morning, he got tea. Breakfast consisted of *poha* (flattened rice) or *suji* (semolina), which was provided at around 7.30 in the morning. By 10.30–11:00 a.m., lunch, consisting of *chappati* (handmade wheat bread) (3), rice (1 bowl), vegetable curry, and *daal* (lentils) was provided. Around 12 noon, only the medical patients received the special medical

---

[10] The traditional Indian system of medicine which is based on the idea of balance in bodily systems and uses diet, herbal treatment, and yogic breathing.

diet: 100 ml of milk, four breads, two bananas, and one sweet lime. After 12 p.m., inmates who had to work in the workshops proceeded for their work.

Although a special diet was given to the prisoners having medical problem, the quality of the food was insipid. The *roti* (handmade wheat bread) was mostly burnt and there was no trace of vegetable in the vegetable curry that they received.

Ram said that there was a prison canteen where inmates could buy foodstuff by exchanging coupons earned by them while working in the prison. He pointed out that he had come across instances where the inmates had smuggled in money from outside, through family members who came to meet them or through the guards.

When asked about the sanitation and the drinking water facility inside the prison, he said that there was one bathroom in one barrack. On an average, each barrack had around 100 inmates. Barrack was a big hall where prisoners were locked, in the afternoon and during the night. There were seven barracks in one circle.[11] Inside every circle, there were four drums for storing water, each drum having a capacity of about 200 litres. Drinking water was stored in three of these drums and the water in the fourth drum was used for washing and cleaning purposes (clothes, utensils, and toilet use). As there was no tap inside the barrack, at night, when they were locked, each inmate had individual bottle in which they stored drinking water for the night. The same water, supplied by the Municipal Corporation, was used both for drinking and washing purposes.

When asked about incidents of violence inside the prison, he said that there had been very few instances. He had seen inmates prepare weapons using stones and fight amongst themselves, but these were very rare occurrences. There was no such abuse from the prison guard. According to him, the prison guards were more interested in performing their duties.

Regarding homosexuality, he said that during his 10 years of stay in the prison, although he had never come across any such situation himself, he had heard a lot about the occurrence of homosexuality. The percentage, according to him, could be in the range of 15–20 %. Usually, the adolescent inmates (18 years to 21 years) were subjected to homosexuality.

Ram had applied to the Inspector General of Prisons (IG), requesting for a transfer to the Central Prison in Kolkata, since his family was in West Bengal. He had been informed that though the IG Maharashtra had approved of his transfer, there was no vacancy in any of the Central Prisons of West Bengal. Ram was eager to get his transfer as it would be easier for his family to meet him. Ram even requested the researcher to talk to the IG regarding his prison transfer. When the Maharashtra IG had come for a visit once, Ram had requested him, in person, for this transfer. During the interaction, the Maharashtra IG had asked him about his working skills. When the IG came to know that he was a jeweller, the IG had said that he might make arrangements so that Ram could start some jewellery-making inside the prison. But it never happened.

---

[11] A separate enclosure with a boundary within the prison; it consists of several barracks where prisoners are housed. Each circle is managed by a jailer.

After release, Ram wanted to send letters to the Supreme Court, Mumbai High Court, and the National Human Rights Commission,[12] informing them about the situation inside the prison. He shared that in the meantime he had collected the addresses of these offices. The very next time, when he would be referred and would go out to the government hospital for treatment, he would get the letters typed, so that he could send those to the aforesaid offices. When asked, how this would be possible, under the supervision of the police guard, he said that he would bribe the guard with some money. On previous occasions, by adopting the same method, he had been able to call up his family from the telephone booth located near the government hospital, when he had gone out for check-up. Although the inmates were frisked before they went out of the prison, he always managed to sneak out some money with himself.

After release, he didn't want to get associated with any organization. He wanted to continue the work of a jeweller, get himself properly treated, and keep his parents happy. He knew that the disease spreads through unprotected sexual contact. He was aware that there was no cure for HIV, but living in a clean environment, intake of adequate amount of water and nutritious diet, light exercise, and keeping the mind free from the worries about the medical condition could go a long way in maintaining a healthy life for a longer period of time. Moreover, there was a need to ensure immediate medical treatment in case of any minor illness.

Case Study III: Ganesh[13]

Ganesh was a 62-year-old elderly man, from Pune district of Maharashtra. He was an illiterate farmer, married, with three children. One of his daughters was married and lived at her in-laws in Mumbai. His two sons had studied till class IX and were engaged in menial occupations for their livelihood (e.g. daily labour in agricultural land). After Ganesh's incarceration, his wife started staying with her parents. Although his mother was no more, his 92-year-old father was still alive. He had five brothers; all of them were illiterate and were engaged in farming within the same village. The land was jointly owned and cultivated by all the siblings together. All brothers used to share the product biannually. However, Ganesh could not assess his share monetarily. Other than chewing of tobacco, he never had any other addiction.

He was convicted, for life, on November 5, 1985, on charges of murder. He had already spent a period of 1 year 4 months and 20 days inside the prison as an undertrial with effect from June 14, 1984, to November 4, 1985.

---

[12] The National Human Rights Commission is an autonomous institution established in October 1993 by the Protection of Human Rights Act, 1993, for the protection and promotion of human rights in India. (Retrieved from www.nhrc.nic.in on June 2, 2014).

[13] Names have been changed. All study participants chose or were assigned a pseudonym.

Around 15 years ago, he used to work in the carpentry section of the prison. He used to cut big logs of wood into small pieces which were then used to make wooden furniture. Once, while he was doing his work, a big nail pierced through his leg and it had to be operated upon. After the operation, a blood clot remained in the affected area. Later, when he was released on furlough,[14] he got the blood clot operated. Due to his medical condition, he returned late to the prison from furlough. He suspected that he got infected with HIV when he was injected during the operation to take out the nail. He felt that the needle used for the injection was not properly sterilized.

In 2002, he developed boils in his hand. The Chief Medical Officer advised him to go for a blood test and referred him to the government hospital. The blood was tested for HIV and it was confirmed that he was HIV positive. He was not aware of HIV and AIDS at that time. Prior to the test, he was not told anything about the nature, purpose, and benefit of the test. He did not pay much heed to it, as he thought that it would be just another disease and the blood was being tested for diagnosis of the same. The test report was communicated by the CMO who informed Ganesh that he was HIV positive.

Ganesh complained of physical ailments and the ineffective medicines in prison.

I suffer from fever and body pain. As if it was not enough, I have also developed piles…as a result of which I cannot even sit properly. I also have these boils. Doctor has prescribed me medicines but nothing works.

Within his term, Ganesh had worked for 12 years. It was only since the last 4 years that he was unable to work because of his ill health.

If I was fit enough to work, I would have worked. But I am weak…I cannot work now. If an inmate living with HIV is capable of working and wants to work, no one stops him.

Ganesh was receiving the special medical diet. However, he was unable to consume the prison food as he was unable to digest it. At around 7 a.m., he got tea and at around 7.30 a.m., approximately 150 ml of milk was served, but it was adulterated with water. The milk was followed by some snacks. The type of snacks varied. Some days it was bread, whereas on other days it was *poha* (flattened rice). The quantity of snacks was approximately 50 gms. The food was not cooked properly and it was very spicy.

Ganesh shared the following issues regarding the availability of water and space inside the prison.

Drinking water is available at the taps in the circle. Each circle consists of almost eight barracks and each barrack has one tap. Inside each barrack, there is one toilet. At night, inmates are locked in the barrack. The three 200 litres drums are filled before the inmates are locked. Inmates convicted for lesser punishment are usually assigned the task of cleaning toilets. Of the three drums, two are for drinking purpose and one is for toilet purpose at night. A barrack, which is around 120 ft in length, houses at least 80 inmates. This space is not sufficient for so many people. Sometimes the number of prisoners increases to 120. During those days, it becomes overcrowded and it is really very difficult to stay within the barrack. Last year, seven ceiling fans have been installed in the barrack where I stay. The prison department provides one bed sheet, one quilt, and one pillow.

---

[14] A prisoner who is sentenced to 5 years or more or rigorous imprisonment but has undergone 3 years of imprisonment excluding remission can be released on furlough.

Ganesh complained about the health-care facility inside the prison.

When I get sick, I am provided with medicines, but none of these medicines work. Sometimes when I have very high fever and feel very weak, I am given injection. Moreover, I cannot eat sufficient food as I find it very spicy.

There were some minor incidents of fighting among the prisoners.

Small fights do happen now and then, but they never get brutal. Moreover, since the guard is around, violent fighting usually does not happen.

When asked about the instance of homosexuality inside the prison, he said that he had only heard of such incidents. He was not sure about the frequency of such incidents.

Ganesh had no problem if others came to know of his HIV-positive status. Some fellow prisoners knew about his status because of the special diet that he received. He himself had also informed many inmates about being HIV positive.

I am an old man now and on top of it I am having this sickness. It is a good thing that other prisoners are becoming aware of this disease through my case. I am going to die, anyway, either of old age or of this disease.

Inside the prison, he was never forcefully segregated because of his HIV-positive status. It was the doctor who decided if an inmate needed to be kept isolated; the patient was never asked whether he wanted to stay in seclusion.

Ganesh did not face any discrimination or stigmatization because of his HIV status.

No one misbehaves with me. Sometimes, it is the illiterate people who are not aware of the disease and tend to misbehave. But, nowadays, everyone is aware of this disease.

Ganesh reported the problem of unavailability of police escort when referred to government hospital.

There is this recurring problem of getting police escort. As a result, often, I am not taken to the government hospital as there are no escorts available. Even when a guard is allotted, by the time I reach the hospital, it is usually past 12. By that time, the OPD section closes and doctors are gone. So, I don't get any medicine. Sometimes, I am given simple painkillers by the prison doctor and not the actual medicine. The allotment of guards for escorting inmates to the government hospital is a major problem for all inmates who are having medical problem and are being referred to the government hospital.

He was aware of HIV and the modes of transmission.

"I have been in the prison for the past 22 years. No outsider has told me anything regarding HIV and AIDS. When I was released on furlough, no one told me anything about the disease. Now I know that proper food should be taken. Medicine should be taken on time, whenever there is some minor illness. One should stay away from bad habits like drinking alcohol and other addictives like ganja (marijuana). If I want to discuss anything related to the disease, I talk to my friends. So far I have not seen anyone to come here and talk about the disease. It's only you…"

He shared his concerns regarding his family. He mentioned that he was in prison since long and was unable to earn because of his age and health condition (inside the prison). Moreover, since his sons could not earn a good living, there was no one to take care of his family. He wished the government would do something for his family.

When asked about his course of action, regarding his treatment after the release, he said that he was not sure. When asked, whether he wanted to get associated with any organization which was working for people living with HIV and AIDS after his release, he expressed his keenness to seek some help for the treatment.

Case Study IV: Prakash[15]

Prakash was 40 years old. Although he was originally from Uttar Pradesh, he was born and brought up in Mumbai. His parents came and settled in Mumbai long ago. His family comprised of his mother, two sisters, and four brothers. One of his sisters was handicapped and one of his brothers was dead. His other sister was married. He was married in the year 1988. He did not have any children. He was 16 years old when his father passed away. Since then, he had been earning a living by taking up small-time jobs like working in hotels etc. Later, he started working as a tailor, along with his brother, before being arrested on the charges of drug peddling. He used to earn around Rs. 1,500 per month. Before incarceration, he had the habit of consuming alcohol occasionally, chewing *pan* (betel leaves), and smoking cigarette. He studied up to Class VII in a Hindi[16] medium school in Mumbai.

He was an undertrial, charged under the Narcotic Drugs and Psychotropic Substances Act (NDPS).[17] His three brothers and wife were arrested on similar charges. His mother and one of his sisters were running the tailoring shop. He had been in the prison for the last 2 years, after being arrested on August 2004 under the NDPS Act. He had a criminal history and had earlier served a sentence, of 5 years of imprisonment, on similar charges under the NDPS Act.

At the time of admission to the prison, he was first taken to the government hospital, for medical examination. He was asked if he was suffering from any health problem. At the prison, during admission, he was asked about his identification mark and his height and weight were recorded.

He believed that he got infected with the disease when he was convicted for the first time. According to him, he was injected with the same syringe that was used to inject other sick inmates. This was because of the ignorance about the disease during that time. He came to know that he was HIV positive when he was arrested for

---

[15] Names have been changed. All study participants chose or were assigned a pseudonym.

[16] Hindi is the official language of India, although English continues to be used as official language along with Hindi.

[17] Narcotic Drugs and Psychotropic Substances Act, 1985, is an Act to consolidate and amend the law relating to narcotic drugs, to make stringent provisions for the control and regulation of operations relating to narcotic drugs and psychotropic substances.

the second time and kept under judicial custody. While in judicial custody, Prakash showed symptoms of TB, after which he met the prison doctor and got the medicines. However, his condition did not improve. The prison doctor referred him to the government hospital. Apart from other tests, the doctor advised the HIV test. Prakash was informed that it was essential to confirm his HIV status as it would make the treatment easier. He agreed to it and his blood was tested for HIV. The doctor told him that he was HIV positive and was also infected with TB. However, the doctor advised Prakash not to worry, as eating nutritious food and following the suggested treatment would help him lead a healthy life. The doctor suggested that Prakash's wife should also get tested for HIV. She was tested HIV negative. After he became aware of his HIV status, he started exercising and practising yoga for fitness.

Prakash underwent treatment at the government hospital and recovered from TB. He was undergoing ART[18] treatment for HIV from the Antiretroviral Therapy Centre of the government hospital. His CD4 count[19] was 143, 6 months ago, and at the time of interview it was 188. He got registered with the ART centre and was given a card, on which the doctor wrote the subsequent appointment date. During every visit, blood check-up, X-ray, and treatment for any other health problem were recommended. But these tests were not done on the same day, as the doctor recommended the required tests to be done in the subsequent visit to the government hospital. However, everything depended on the availability of the guards. It used to take a minimum of 15 days to get a guard as an escort to the government hospital, thus delaying the receipt of the test reports. If he went to the CMO of the prison and requested him to make arrangements for his upcoming appointment at the government hospital, the CMO used to write his name in the diary. This was then sent to the prison superintendent, who arranged for the guards depending upon the number of inmates who had been referred by the prison doctor to the government hospital.

---

[18] Standard antiretroviral therapy (ART) consists of the combination of at least three antiretroviral (ARV) drugs to maximally suppress the HIV virus and stop the progression of HIV disease. Huge reductions have been seen in rates of death and suffering when use is made of a potent ARV regimen, particularly in early stages of the disease. Retrieved from http://www.who.int/hiv/topics/treatment/en/ on July 2, 2014.

[19] The CD4 count is done to measure the strength of the immune system if someone is diagnosed with HIV infection and to examine how far HIV disease has advanced. CD4 cells are a type of white blood cells, also known as a t-cell. The cells that HIV infects are most often CD4 cells. With HIV infection, the DNA of the virus becomes part of the CD4 cell. Paradoxically, when CD4 cells multiply as an immune response to the infection, they also make more replications of the virus. As the virus progresses, the body makes fewer CD4 cells, while copies of the virus proliferate. A person with fewer than 200 CD4 cells is considered to have AIDS (Castro et al. 1992). The CD4 count is also used to identify possible health problems for which the patient may be at risk and to determine which medications might be helpful. The CD4 count is most useful when it is compared with the count obtained from an earlier test. In general, the CD4 count goes down as HIV disease progresses. According to public health guidelines, preventive therapy should be started when an HIV-positive person who has no symptoms registers a CD4 count under 200. (Retrieved from http://labtestsonline.org/understanding/analytes/cd4/tab/test on June 12, 2014).

If he requested four to five times a week, chances were he might get the guard once. The test reports were handed over to him when he finally managed to visit the hospital. Inside the prison, no medical treatment was available for inmates living with HIV. The latest advice of the doctor of the government hospital was to continue his medicines regularly and visit once a month for check-up. However, reaching the government hospital depended on the availability of guards. According to him, during his treatment for TB, his treatment got discontinued as he could not reach the hospital on the next due date because of the non-availability of guards.

According to Prakash, in case of people living with HIV, medicines required for treatment of even simple ailments like fever were different from those required for treating those who were not HIV positive.

> Inside the jail, there is no provision for treatment. Even for a simple ailment like indigestion, medicines effective for other inmates have no effect on HIV positive people.

Prakash was receiving medical diet meant for the HIV-positive patients in the prison. However, the quality of the food was not good. Food was spicy and not fit for consumption. He was fortunate enough to get permission to have home-cooked food twice a day—at 12 p.m. and around 3 p.m. Court order for home-cooked food could be obtained by submitting an application along with the medical certificate. Either the inmate or any other relative of the inmate could directly apply to the magistrate for the same, without appointing any advocate. Prakash asked his sister to get the permission when she visited him in the prison. When he used to take prison food, he was receiving the special medical diet, which consisted of 250 ml of milk and bread in addition to the normal diet. He said that the milk was adulterated. Prakash was put up in a barrack in the hospital ward. It was a 15 by 15 feet room, had two fans, and one toilet. According to him, the barrack in which he was staying was much better than those inside the circles. This he knew, as initially he was kept in one of those circles.

On the role of NGOs, he said that the NGOs working in the prison generally provided counselling services for the prison inmates living with HIV. He felt that those NGOs who were interested to work inside the prison for the treatment of prisoners living with HIV should be granted permission for the same by the prison administration.

He was of the opinion that prevalence of homosexuality inside the prison might be one percent. He felt that homosexuality was more prevalent in prisons where long-term convicts were lodged. In overcrowded prisons, where most of the inmates were undertrials, incidents of homosexuality couldn't take place due to the lack of privacy.

Although the inmates living with HIV were normally not lodged in separate barracks on the grounds of their HIV status, if a prison inmate living with HIV suffered from any contagious disease, which might spread to other healthy prisoners, he was lodged in a separate ward.

Space was a problem in the prison. In a 20 by 20 feet room, as many as 20 inmates were cramped together.

According to him, if free voluntary testing was offered inside the prison, guaranteeing confidentiality, as many as 90 % of the inmates would be willing to come forward for voluntary testing.

He said that if he had been outside the prison, he would have ensured regular and proper treatment for himself at the government hospital. He lamented that getting police escort to the court, for the hearing of his case, was a problem, too. His case was running since the last 8 months. Sometimes, when guards were available for escort, either the judge or the prosecutor would be absent, thus delaying the hearing of his case.

Prakash explained the procedure of receiving medical treatment in the following words:

> When I was ill, I could meet the doctor since my barrack is in the hospital ward. At night, there is a nursing orderly who attends to inmates who are sick and require help. On the other hand, if an inmate from the circle wants to meet the doctor, he has to enter his name in the register kept at the hospital gate and then wait for his call. Inmates can also meet the doctor when the prison doctor is doing rounds. The doctors do not examine the inmates regularly. If an inmate falls sick and meets the doctor, the doctor prescribes the treatment and medicine or refers him to the government hospital, if required. Accordingly, his name is put in a diary and the diary goes to the prison superintendent, who signs and sends the list and requirement of police guard to the police department, which then arranges for police escort for the prisoners.

No visiting doctor or specialist came to the prison. He never faced any problem with the prison doctors and the paramedical staff. The attitude of the doctors and other prisoners towards him was normal. The major problem he faced was that of unavailability of guard escorts to visit the government hospital.

The OPD at the government hospital closed at 12 p.m. Sometimes, even when guard was allotted to him, he could only reach the government hospital after 12 p.m. So, there were instances when he had to come back without meeting the doctor. Medicines were provided free of cost, both in prison and in the government hospital. The prisoner living with HIV and AIDS was hospitalized only when he was seriously ill. There were many instances when the inmates faked sickness so that they could go out of the prison to the government hospital.

Sometimes, the guards who escorted Prakash to the Government hospital asked about his disease. When Prakash shared that he was HIV positive, some of them got frightened. He cited a day when after hearing that Prakash was HIV positive, the guard left his hand and clutched his shirt collar. According to Prakash, people who were educated and knew about the disease behaved in a rude manner; whereas people who were illiterate did not show much concern.

When asked about the organizations working inside the prison on HIV and AIDS, Prakash said that the previous month an organization visited the prison and conducted dental check-up camp. He mentioned about an organization which worked in the prison for de-addiction and occasionally provided counselling services for inmates living with HIV and AIDS. His family, wife, and people living in his neighbourhood were aware that he was HIV positive. Inside the prison, the fellow prisoners knew about his HIV status. He did not have any problem with other people being aware of his HIV-positive status. Medical records and pathological reports were directly handed over to him, which he gave to the prison doctor. Some time back, he applied for bail on the grounds of being HIV positive. The court ordered for the confirmation of his HIV-positive status and he was tested again at the government hospital. The report of his HIV-positive status was directly sent to the court from the government hospital.

He was not asked to stay separate because of his HIV-positive status. Prakash mentioned that in order to maintain a normal healthy life, he was required to eat healthy food, maintain hygiene, and stay away from addictions of all types. Regarding the preventive measures, he said that he needed to use condoms.

Case Study V: Shyam[20]

He was 26 years old and hailed from Kishanganj district of Bihar. He ran away from home in the year 1993 as he was scolded and beaten up by his parents. He came looking for work in Mumbai. His first job was washing utensils in hotels. After that, he worked as a construction labourer at construction sites. Subsequently, he learnt tailoring (in 3 months) and started earning Rs. 1,500–2,000 per month. It was then that his three brothers followed him to Mumbai and they, together, opened a tailoring shop and started earning Rs. 6,000–10,000 per month, collectively. It was during this time that he developed the habit of visiting brothels. He didn't have any addictions like smoking or drinking because he believed that such habits would make him prone to contract TB. At the time of admission in the prison as an undertrial, there was no medical check-up. After spending 3 months as an undertrial, he was out of prison on bail for 19 months. Later, he was convicted in a kidnapping case and sentenced for 3 years and 4 months. Before admission in the prison after conviction, he was taken to the government hospital, where he was asked by the doctor if he had any physical problem. Since Shyam felt perfectly well and did not know of any physical ailment that he was suffering from, he shared the same with the doctor. After a month, Shyam was transferred to another prison, where he was serving his sentence.

At home, he never went to school as he hated studies. His family consisted of father, mother, wife, and one child. They were residing at his home in Bihar. He got married in 2001. His father was a businessman who sold seeds of various vegetables and his brother was a tailor. At the time of his marriage, he did not have any information about HIV and AIDS.

---

[20] Names have been changed. All study participants chose or were assigned a pseudonym.

While serving his sentence, he came to know that he was HIV positive. He developed boils and none of the medicines prescribed by the prison doctor were found to be effective. The prison doctor referred him to the government hospital, where he was advised to go for an HIV test. Shyam, when asked whether he had any objection to the blood test, expressed his willingness. The doctor also explained to him in detail about HIV and the reason for which the test was necessary. His blood report, positive, was communicated to him by the doctor at the government hospital.

> After the test, I was put in a single room, separately. The doctor said that if I stay with other inmates they might develop the same skin infection. I don't like to stay separate. I like it better in the cell where I have stayed for 5 months and where I can interact with other inmates.

Shyam was referred to the government hospital at Mumbai, which is the referral hospital for prison inmates living with HIV. He was transferred to the prison in Mumbai for this purpose. His CD4 count was conducted in the referral hospital. Though no further treatment was recommended, he was advised to visit the ART Centre on a subsequent date.

His wife had not been tested for HIV. His family was not aware of his HIV status. According to him, if they came to know that he was living with HIV, they would disown him. After his release from the prison, he would get his wife and child tested.

Shyam mentioned that in the prison where he was initially lodged, there was no problem of overcrowding and the food served was of better quality than that served in the prison where he was lodged at the time of interview. He shared the following regarding the poor quality of food which was being served in the prison:

> Though different sabjis (vegetable curries) are served on different days, the food is not palatable. The chapattis are not properly cooked and vegetables are not fit for consumption. I am forced to eat the uncooked food to stay alive. Do I really deserve this kind of treatment?

According to Shyam, sometimes even better space could be arranged inside the circle.

> Space poses a major problem for the inmates. Inside the circle, it is difficult even to get enough space to sleep properly. In exchange of money or sex, one can manage even to get a better place to sleep. Every Saturday, one or more inmates are released. The warder, thus, can manage better space in exchange of money.

Shyam was put up in the hospital ward.

> This barrack is better still. The room is around 15/15 ft, accommodating 14–15 inmates on an average. However, still, the space is insufficient and suffocative. In other circles, the situation is worse. People are more and the space is limited.

When asked about his views regarding the prison medical services, he said that there was no medical facility inside the prison. There was no provision for special doctor to cater to the inmates who were living with HIV or for those suffering from TB. Shyam felt that there should be a special doctor who would visit the prison once in a week or fortnight for inmates living with HIV. There could be many prisoners who did not know that they were HIV positive. There were many inmates who did not want to disclose their HIV-positive status, fearing stigma. So, if a special doctor came inside the prison for check-ups, then inmates might come forward for testing.

In the prison, when someone falls sick, he goes to the prison doctor who provides medicines. The prison doctor comes every day. He further explained that if the medicine doesn't work and the condition of the patient deteriorates, then he is referred to the government hospital.

> One undertrial prisoner, who was HIV positive, was in a critical condition. He was unable to eat anything. He was not even able to go to the toilet. He was taken to the government hospital where he died. One special doctor for HIV positive inmates is essential.

At the time of admission in the prison, he had no information on HIV and AIDS. Few prisoners had explained to him, later, about how HIV spreads. Shyam came to know, in detail, about HIV and AIDS when he was detected HIV positive and the doctor explained to him the details of the disease.

> It spreads through sharing infected blade meant for shaving. If health problems continue to increase and the usual medicines do not work, then it is a symptom of HIV. HIV spreads through unprotected sex with multiple partners and from infected mother to the child. The doctor also told me that if I take medicines regularly and lead a healthy life it is possible to live longer. I will spread the message about HIV.

When asked, regarding homosexual activities inside the prison, he said that though he himself had not encountered any such incident, he had heard about it and estimated the occurrence to be around 5 %.

He did not come across any organization which had come to visit the prison to discuss or work on HIV.

Other inmates in the barrack knew that he was HIV positive.

> They might have come to know from the special medical diet that I receive. I did not inform my family that I am HIV positive as I know that this information will only cause tension. Though the medical reports remain with the prison doctor, other medical staff might also know that I am HIV positive. I told the prison superintendent, once, that I am HIV positive, when he came for a round inside the circle, hoping that my treatment will start. If I had done this test before and had appealed in the court, my punishment tenure might have been less on the grounds of being HIV positive.

He described the living space where he was lodged.

> The barrack where I am put up, houses five HIV positive inmates. Others include asthma patients, handicapped and weak inmates or those arrested for drug abuse. They all are lodged in this barrack. This barrack is in the hospital ward and we all are sick people. So in case of any health problem we can easily visit the doctor.

> In each circle there are approximately ten barracks. The barrack, in which I am staying, is smaller and is approximately 15 by 15 ft. There is one latrine at the corner of the barrack.

One TV is provided inside the barrack. There are two taps for drinking water in the circle. Though, earlier there was scarcity of water, it has been resolved.

After release, he wanted to continue the treatment if it started during his stay in the prison. If the treatment didn't start in prison, he would get associated with organizations helping people living with HIV and AIDS, after release.

At the end of the interview, he again insisted for a special doctor. This, he suggested, would also solve the problem of allotment of guards, which was a major problem, since for one inmate a minimum of two to a maximum of 12 guards were required, depending on the nature of crime committed by the inmate. If the special doctor visited regularly then there would be no gap in the treatment. The doctor would at least take blood sample for check-up and could get medicines inside the prison so that the treatment could continue uninterrupted. Furthermore, a patient would be referred to the government hospital only when he needed to be admitted.

Case Study VI: Anil[21]

Anil was a 38 years old inmate, originally from Banaras (Varanasi), Uttar Pradesh, who came to Mumbai 17 years back. He was born and brought up at Banaras, where he was residing with his paternal uncle's family. In Mumbai, he was staying with his father, mother, wife, and his three children. His father had a furniture shop. His daughter was in Class IV, one son in Class III, and the other in kindergarten. He had completed his Bachelors in Science with physics, chemistry, and mathematics from Banaras Hindu University. He got admission in National Defence Academy. It was during his 6 months training period, there, when his father expired. He had to leave the course and start his own electronics business to earn a living. He was involved in buying, selling, and repairing of electronic goods on contract basis with the Pawan Hans refinery owned by the Oil and Natural Gas Commission. He used to earn Rs. 10,000–15,000 per month. In 1998, he was arrested under the Narcotic Drugs and Psychotropic Substances Act and was kept as a detenue[22] for 2 years. He was convicted in August 2000 and sentenced for 10 years.

During his detention, he suffered from severe food poisoning, for which he was administered an injection. According to him, he was injected with the same needle which was used to inject an inmate living with HIV, without proper sterilization. Later, a nursing staff revealed this fact to him. In those days (1998–1999), single- use/disposable syringes were not used; usually, the same syringes were used after sterilizing them in hot water. Most of the times, the needles were not properly sterilized. The water was boiled in the morning and the same water was used throughout the day.

---

[21] Name has been changed. All study participants chose or were assigned a pseudonym.

[22] An accused who is detained and is under trial for an alleged crime.

After getting infected, within a year he started losing weight and frequently started to suffer from flu. He was referred to the government hospital for check-up and was diagnosed with malaria. During his treatment for malaria, he was also suggested to get the blood tested for HIV. He was told about the nature of the test and was asked if he was willing to get himself tested. He gave his consent and his test result was positive. The doctor started explaining him about the implications of having HIV. Considering this discussion unnecessary, he asked the doctor to come to the point and share the result. After coming to know that he was HIV positive, Anil asked his wife to get tested for HIV. His wife was tested negative.

According to him, even if one blade contained ten microns of infected blood, the virus might get transmitted if used by another uninfected person. He expressed deep frustration by saying that he did not deserve to be in this condition. He was already suffering, being in the prison, and in addition to that he developed the deadly disease only due to the negligence of the prison staff. He had to sell his shop and his family had to shift to a cheaper accommodation. He said that he would have committed suicide, long back, had his family not been there.

He was registered with the Antiretroviral Therapy (ART) Centre of J. J. Hospital, the referral hospital, in Mumbai. This ART Centre provided treatment and conducted CD4 count of people living with HIV. The procedure for getting a transfer to the prison in Mumbai was very cumbersome.

Since there was no ART centre at Nasik Government Hospital, any inmate lodged in the prison in Nasik, who needed ART, had to be referred to J. J. Hospital, Mumbai, which had an ART centre. For this, an inmate needed to be transferred from the prison in Nasik to the prison in Mumbai. Anil explains the process of transfer in the following words:

> When the doctor of Nasik prison refers an inmate to J. J. Hospital, it is practically not possible to visit the J. J. Hospital in Mumbai, as it is 5 hours journey, by road, from Nasik. Also, a convict prisoner has to seek permission from the concerned Deputy Inspector General of Prisons (DIG), who in turn refers the case to Mumbai DIG. Only when the Mumbai DIG gives his permission, the inmate can be transferred to Mumbai Central Prison from Nasik.

Anil was advised to visit the referral hospital, for regular check-up. But since the process of transfer took a long time, his treatment got interrupted for months together and he ran out of medicines. Presently, he was being treated for TB in J. J. Hospital. Although the medicine was given and he was asked to visit the hospital regularly for checkup, it was practically not possible due to non-availability of guards.

Anil had undergone appendicitis operation in the government hospital of the city where he was initially lodged. He felt that adequate medicines were not available in that hospital. Also, the doctors were very rude. It was a general tendency of the doctors to behave rudely with prisoners and he was no exception.

The quality of food in the prison was very bad and it was very spicy. Although milk and eggs were given as a special diet, milk was always adulterated with water. Anil had the experience of staying in two prisons. In both the prisons he had been receiving medical diet as prescribed by the doctors. As part of the normal diet, he used to get one banana and 150 ml of milk. In one of the prisons, two eggs were also served. In the morning, around 8 a.m., he was given 200 ml of milk and bread. Around 11 a.m., he was given one bowl of rice, three *chappatis* (handmade wheat bread), one bowl of *daal* (lentils), and vegetable curry. The dinner consisted of the same menu, with a change in the vegetable curry. Though he was not supposed to eat spicy food, he had no other option but to eat it.

He noticed some differences in both the prisons where he was lodged. In one prison, he was put up in a separate ward, called 'HIV ward', where other sick inmates were kept. Overcrowding was a terrible problem in the barrack. In the other prison, there was no issue of overcrowding.

In one of the prisons, sometimes, the police guards who escorted him to the government hospital behaved rudely with him. In the other prison as well, the allotment of police escort was a huge problem. Fortunately, if escort was allotted and he reached hospital, it was already past 12 in the afternoon and the OPD was closed. He had to come back without any treatment. Even if he was able to meet the doctor, he did not receive any treatment as the doctor scheduled another appointment, on a subsequent day, after check-up. Again, getting a police guard for the next appointment was a problem. So, treatment was not regular and there was a gap in the treatment.

When asked, if there was any situation inside the prison where HIV might get transmitted through activities like homosexuality, Anil said that he didn't experience any such incident but had heard about it. According to him, based on whatever he had heard, prevalence of homosexuality might be around 5–10 % inside the prison.

Anil informed that he had not come across anyone who had provided him with information or education on HIV and AIDS inside the prison. He came to know about HIV and AIDS from the newspapers. He also practised yoga to stay fit.

He expressed that staying at Nasik made it very difficult to continue ART, as he was required to meet the doctor every month and for that he needed to apply for permission to get transferred to the prison in Mumbai. This was a major problem.

After release, he would continue his treatment at the referral hospital. He would take medicines regularly, attend appointments for check-up on the scheduled dates, and would ensure that there was no gap in the treatment. Apart from this, he would have nutritious food, as suggested by the doctor. He was eager to work on HIV and AIDS, both, to receive help and help any organization working on HIV and AIDS.

Case Study VII: Shiv[23]

Shiv hailed from Deoaria, Uttar Pradesh, and was 35 years old. He had three sisters and two brothers. All his sisters were married and his younger brother was a farmer in the village. His parents were staying with his younger brother after he was

---

[23] Name has been changed. All study participants chose or were assigned a pseudonym.

incarcerated. His elder brother was working as a cook in Delhi and was married, with four children. He didn't have any kind of addiction when he was in his native place. He studied till tenth standard, after which he dropped out from school, as he was not interested in studies.

In 1989, when he was 20 years old, he came to Mumbai accompanying another person from his village. He was successful in finding a job as a security guard within 2 months of his arrival to the city. He took leave, and went home, for 5 months, before the serial bomb blasts in Mumbai in 1993.[24] He came back and resumed his duty. He was arrested for possession of *charas* (a form of cannabis), along with his fellow villager who was living with him in the same room. He was convicted and sentenced to ten and a half years of imprisonment under NDPS Act on March 1997. He was serving the last month of his sentence at the time of the interview.

During his stay in the prison, in the year 2000, once, while playing football, his leg was injured. The prison doctor administered injection for his treatment. However, the pain in his leg persisted and he was advised to take painkillers twice a day. During this period, he was not aware of HIV and AIDS. When his condition did not improve, he was referred to the government hospital where the doctor referred him to J. J. Hospital in Mumbai for further treatment. Hence he was shifted to the prison in Mumbai. The doctors at the referral hospital advised him to get his blood tested for HIV. Prior to the test, Shiv was told about the nature and purpose of the blood test. He was explained about HIV. He was told that since the medicines for the minor leg injury were ineffective, it was necessary for him to get the HIV test done. Shiv agreed, as he, too, wanted to get rid of the disease. The blood reports were positive and the doctors at the referral hospital told Shiv that he was HIV positive. They explained to him the implications of having the disease. He was suggested to take extreme care of himself and precautions. He was advised that if he took adequate care of himself, with proper food and nutrition, it was possible for him to live a normal healthy life.

After he was tested positive for HIV, he was sent back to the prison where he was initially lodged. He was advised medical diet. As part of the medical diet, Shiv used to receive 200 ml of milk and banana in addition to the normal diet. At around 8 in the morning, he used to get 200 ml of milk and bread. At around 11 a.m., he was given lunch, which consisted of one bowl of rice, three *chapattis* (handmade wheat bread), one vegetable curry, and one bowl of *daal* (lentils). The same menu was served for dinner, only with a change in the type of vegetable curry. He said that the quality of the food was not good and that the milk was adulterated with water. The food was spicy and difficult to digest.

He said that in case of any health problem, he could approach any Medical Officer, who, if required, could refer him to the government hospital. In case, he had to be referred to the government hospital, the prison doctor wrote to the superinten-

---

[24] The name given to the 13 serial explosions that took place in Mumbai on Friday, March 12, 1993.

dent of the prison for permission. The superintendent arranged the police guard who could escort him to the Government Hospital. However, there was a huge problem in allotment of police escort. So, even if the doctor referred him to the Government Hospital, until he was allotted guard(s), he could not go to the Government Hospital for the required check-up. Shiv was referred to the referral hospital in Mumbai for CD4 count test.

Shiv shared his experiences, of being lodged in two prisons. He said that in one prison, people were just huddled together. He was put up in a barrack in the hospital ward where other sick people were also lodged. The number of undertrial prisoners was more. Sometimes the number of inmates in the barrack increased, which made the place congested.

Shiv volunteered for an experiment conducted by NARI for a drug on HIV. He felt that NARI had thorough knowledge about HIV treatment. Also, the doctors at NARI treated the people living with HIV like any other patient. He also mentioned about a doctor in the referral hospital who was kind and who treated him well. But the doctors in Government Hospital treated him very badly. He further elaborated that the people (doctors and other medical staff in the hospital) did not even touch him.

He wanted to get transferred to any prison in Mumbai or Thane so that he could get regular medical treatment, which was not possible, staying in Nasik, as it was far away from J. J. Hospital. Also, the process to get permission for prison transfer was lengthy and included getting permission from Deputy Inspector General (DIG) of Prisons, both of Aurangabad and Mumbai, which was very complicated. Even when he was transferred to the prison in Mumbai, it was not always possible to visit the referral hospital. Shiv explained that unless he was allotted guard as escort, he could not be sent to the referral hospital for treatment. So, he had to wait, even when he was in Mumbai, where he was supposed to get regular medical treatment.

Regarding homosexuality, he said that he had never experienced any such incident but had heard about it in the prison. He had no issues, with other people coming to know of his HIV status. He himself was ready to disclose that he was HIV positive.

He said that the doctors in the prison were aware of his HIV status. This was because it was the doctor who kept his medical record. Some fellow prisoners were also aware that he was living with HIV because of the medical diet that he received. He also added that the prisoners did not show any hatred towards any inmate who was living with HIV.

After release, Shiv wanted to continue treatment. He said that in the prison he was getting free treatment, but when released, he would like to get himself treated at a private hospital. After release, he would get married to a lady who was HIV positive and when his wife would get pregnant, he would make her undergo treatment. He knew that through proper medication during pregnancy, it was possible to prevent HIV from getting transmitted from mother to the child.

He was also aware of the law, which permitted early release for people suffering from incurable diseases.

After his release, Shiv wanted to get associated with an organization and spread the message about HIV and AIDS. Post-release, he would take precautions during any sexual act. He felt that proper treatment should be provided to people living with HIV and AIDS.

Cases at a Glance

The above seven case studies have been structured as narratives, after the initial data collected from the field. Table 3.1 highlights the cases at a glance.

Table 3.1 Cases at a glance…

Cases	Age (in years)	Whether migrant	Occupation prior to incarceration	Average income (per month)	History of drug abuse	Cause of HIV infection	Educational background
Raja	35	No	Salesman	Rs. 2,000	No	Unprotected sex with multiple partners	Standard Ninth
Ram	29	Yes	Jeweller	Rs. 7,000	No	-do-	Standard Fourth
Ganesh	62	No	Farmer	Not sure	No	Non-sterilized needle impregnation during treatment while in prison	Illiterate
Prakash	40	No	Tailor	Rs. 1,500	No	-do-	Standard Seventh
Shyam	26	Yes	Tailor	Rs. 10, 000	No	Unprotected sex with multiple partners	Illiterate
Anil	38	Yes	Business	Rs. 10,000–15,000	No	Non-sterilized needle impregnation during treatment while in prison	Graduate (BSc)
Shiv	35	Yes	Security guard	Rs. 2,000	No	Unprotected sex with multiple partners	Standard Tenth

Socio-economic Situation of the Inmates Living with HIV

Age

Analysis of the seven individual cases shows that the age of six inmates living with HIV can be clustered within the age group of 25–40 years. These were their ages at the time of the interview. It can be assumed that they got infected with the virus, more than 3–5 years back, when they were younger—maybe, around 20–35 years old. It has been observed that people between the ages of 18–35 are less likely to be in monogamous relationships and have wider sexual network. So they are more likely to contract HIV and other sexually transmitted infections (STIs) (HIV/AIDS among Youth 2008). Although in this study, none of the inmates shared having any sexually transmitted infection, it cannot be negated that all six inmates were in an age group vulnerable to contract HIV.

Educational Background

Education plays an important role in widening the knowledge base and developing a rational outlook towards life. In the context of HIV and AIDS, HIV education programmes may not reach the uneducated and illiterate people, thus causing their lower levels of HIV and AIDS knowledge (Goyer 2003). The study indicates that two inmates were illiterate and four couldn't cross the primary level of school education. All the seven inmates, who contracted HIV, had bare minimum educational qualification, except for one inmate who had completed his graduation. Six of the inmates did not have any information about HIV and AIDS until they were detected with HIV. This scenario, somehow, confirms the notion that lower level of education determines the level of knowledge and awareness regarding HIV and AIDS.

Employment and Occupation Status

Before being incarcerated, all seven inmates were employed in different kinds of occupations.

Income (Per Month)

Two inmates were earning a salary of around Rs. 10, 000 and the earning of four inmates was below Rs. 10,000. One inmate was not sure about his income in monetary terms.

Incarceration History

Six inmates were convicts and one was an undertrial. Three inmates were convicted for murder and were serving life imprisonment. Raja had served 9 years and was in the tenth year of his imprisonment at the time of interview. Ram was serving his seventh year and Ganesh was in his twenty-second year of imprisonment. Prakash and Anil were under charges of NDPS Act. While Anil and Shiv were already convicted for 10 years and ten and half years, respectively, Prakash was an undertrial, awaiting the court verdict. Only Prakash was a habitual offender, who was convicted, even before, under the same charges. Shyam was convicted for kidnapping and had 6 more months of the sentence to be served.

Implications of Socio-economic Situation

The socio-economic situation of the seven inmates indicates that six out of seven inmates were in their middle age, when they contracted the virus. Although everyone was employed prior to incarceration, six of them were having less education and less income. Thus, while two inmates can be categorized under the middle-income group, others belonged to the lower income group. Poverty and illiteracy could be a major reason for lower access to health education, preventive measures for HIV and AIDS, and medical care. This results in an increased risk of contracting HIV. This is further evident from the fact that six inmates did not have any information regarding HIV and AIDS before being incarcerated. Only one inmate, who was a science graduate, knew about HIV and AIDS even before he developed the symptoms. Furthermore, three inmates were in the prison on the charges of NDPS. Though they denied having injected any drug, the fact that low socio-economic status is related to drug use and high-risk sexual activity cannot be negated. As mentioned by Braithwaite et al. (1996), in low socio-economic communities, young people are aware of drug availability and of the harsher elements of society. Drug use is also an escape from the immediate and harsh realities of the society. Besides, four inmates were involved in high-risk behaviour (unprotected sex with multiple partners), which was the cause of contracting the virus. These are the people who had low income. It may be said that low income may lead to high-risk sexual behaviour, leading to a higher risk of contracting HIV. Thus, it seems that low socio-economic status has strong relation with drug use and hypersexual activity.

Marital Status

Five inmates were married, of which four had children. Only one inmate had gone out of the prison on furlough. However, by the time of his release on furlough, he was aware that he was HIV positive and knew about the precautions to be taken so as to prevent the spread of the disease. However, at the time of his release on furlough, no one from the prison discussed with him the preventive measures to be taken. Two inmates reported that after they came to know that they were HIV positive, they asked their wives to get tested for HIV and their wives were found to be HIV negative. Two inmates came to know that they were HIV positive while they were inside the prison and didn't ask their wives to go for the HIV test. Both of them had a history of high-risk behaviour, before being incarcerated. One of them didn't even disclose his HIV status to his wife. There is a chance that both their wives may also be infected with HIV.

Migrant/Non-migrant

Among the seven people interviewed, four were migrants from other states to Maharashtra. They left home and settled in Mumbai in search of a better livelihood. Three inmates contracted the disease through unprotected sexual contact. However, none of them reported of any history of injecting drug abuse. Migration may be a factor that might have facilitated sexual contact with multiple partners, one of the high-risk behaviours.

History of Drug and Alcohol Use

Three inmates were arrested under NDPS Act. All of them negated any habit of drug abuse, in general, and injecting drug use, in particular. However, they mentioned that they occasionally consumed alcohol. Two inmates, though not convicted under the same Act, did mention about occasional drinking habit prior to incarceration.

High-Risk Behaviour Prior to Incarceration

Four inmates contracted the disease through unprotected sexual contact with multiple partners before incarceration. However, none of them reported sex in exchange of drugs or needle-sharing for injecting drug. These high-risk behaviours, before incarceration, place prisoners at higher risk of HIV. One inmate was released on furlough and another was an undertrial, which means that these two inmates were in and out of the prison more often than the convicts. Released prisoners resume high-risk behaviour like unprotected sex and drug abuse (Dolan & Larney 2010) and incarcerated persons report more IDU and unsafe sexual practices than the general population (Glaser & Greifinger 1993). Literature also suggests that formerly incarcerated individuals frequently engage in unsafe sex with multiple partners

Table 3.2 Knowledge of inmates regarding prevalence of disease

Name	Year in which inmate came to know that he is HIV positive	Year of admission in prison as undertrial	Year of admission in prison as convict
Raja	2004	1997	2000
Ram	2003	1996	1999
Ganesh	2002	1984	1985
Prakash	2004	2004	NA
Shyam	2006	2003	2004
Anil	1999	1998	2000
Shiv	2000	1993	1997

(Hudson et al. 2011). As mentioned by Goyer (2003), these behaviours are regardless of environmental factors or social exclusion. Under the influence of drugs, people may indulge in other high-risk behaviours, including high-risk sexual activity and needle-sharing for injecting drug. As there are no effective intervention programmes and policies, there is a possibility that this type of pre-incarceration behaviour might continue even after incarceration or resume after release from prison.

Although none of the inmates agreed to a history of injecting drug use, it is observed in a study, conducted in 1997–2000, that around 8 % of individuals imprisoned in Tihar Jail in Delhi were drug users and 63 % inmates in Delhi, Mumbai, and Punjab prison reported drug use before incarceration (Dolan & Larney 2010). Studies reveal that people who are drug users also land up in prison (UNODC 2002).

Knowledge of the Prevalence of the Disease

From Table 3.2, it is evident that all the seven inmates came to know that they were HIV positive only after coming to the prison, when visible symptoms, like skin disease etc., began to appear, and the common corresponding medicines, available at the prison, proved ineffective.

Cause of HIV

Four inmates contracted the disease as a result of unprotected sex with multiple sexual partners. The other three inmates reported to have contracted the disease when they were injected with non-sterilized needles, during treatment, while in prison. While two inmates admitted that it was due to ignorance, regarding the disease during the 1990s, that the same needles were used for injecting medicines without proper sterilization, one inmate mentioned that it was because of negligence of the prison medical staff.

Knowledge and Awareness of HIV and AIDS

All seven inmates appeared to have fair knowledge and awareness regarding the preventive aspects of HIV. Only one inmate, who was a science graduate, knew about HIV and AIDS prior to incarceration. The rest of the six inmates came to know about the details, regarding HIV and AIDS, only after incarceration when they developed opportunistic infections.

Raja also mentioned about medicines for people living with HIV. He was not diagnosed with AIDS. It was not clear to him that medicines can only be prescribed for opportunistic infections and not particularly for HIV.

Anil seemed to be quite knowledgeable regarding the disease. Not only was he aware of the causative and preventive factors of HIV and AIDS, he also mentioned the minimum amount of infected blood that was capable of transmitting the virus.

Ram, Prakash, and Shiv were aware of HIV and AIDS——the mode of transmission and prevention and measures that could be adopted in order to stay healthy for a longer period of time.

Source of Information on HIV and AIDS

Three inmates mentioned TV and newspaper as the source of information. Ram also reported collecting newspaper cuttings of reports on HIV and AIDS. He also mentioned about few posters on HIV and AIDS which were on display in the prison hospital ward. Only one inmate shared that his source of information was from the pre-test and post-test HIV counselling. Some came to know from other inmates living with HIV.

Post-release Plans

Three inmates expressed their desire to get associated with voluntary organization for continuation of their treatment. Two inmates wanted to continue their treatment at the government hospital, post-release. One inmate didn't want to get attached to any NGO and wanted to continue his profession. One inmate was 'not sure' about his future and couldn't specify any post-release plan. Another inmate wanted to get married and settle down. He also wanted to get associated with an organization, to spread the message about HIV and AIDS. He wanted to resume his treatment at a private hospital. Two inmates specifically mentioned of maintaining a healthy lifestyle.

Conclusion

The present analysis, covering several dimensions of social and economic background of the inmate population, reveals that majority of inmates were convicts, married, and in the age group of 25–40 years. Majority of the inmates, living with HIV and AIDS, engaged in high-risk sexual behaviour before imprisonment. The chapter also throws light on the extent of knowledge and information regarding HIV and AIDS and the source of information regarding the same. The next chapter discusses the experiences of prison inmates living with HIV.

Chapter 4
Experiences of Prison Inmates Living with HIV

Prisons have been referred to as total institutions (Goffman 1961) where prisoners undergo a process of prisonization. Prison environment is characterized by a specific set of morals, rules, laws, social relations, patterns of behaviour, and problems. Prisonization refers to adjusting to this prison environment. In total institutions, each member of the group is treated alike and is required to do similar things together. All activities are tightly scheduled and are planned under the same central authority. Total institutions are also characterized by the 'inmate world' and the 'staff world', each having distinguished characteristics. While the self-esteem of the inmate is challenged in the 'inmate world' due to several factors (Goffman 1961), the staff in the 'staff world' faces 'burnout', chronic stress, and tension (Fox 1983). The prison environment deprives the inmates of certain basic needs, described as the 'pains of imprisonment' by Graham Sykes (1958) in his study titled 'The Society of Captives'. The pains of imprisonment include loss of liberty, access to goods and services, heterosexual relationships, and autonomy. Security affects an inmate's attitude, self-image, values, and behaviour, and a unique culture called the 'inmate code' develops. This is referred to as the deprivation model which explains that the behaviour of an inmate changes inside the prison as a result of prisonization process (Gillespie 2005; Krebs 2002). In contrast to the deprivation model, the importation model (Schrag 1961) holds that inmate behaviour is explained by experiences of the inmate before incarceration which is imported into the prison from the outside world (Thomas & Cage 1977). In the context of HIV and AIDS, certain behaviours and experiences of the inmates may be influenced by the above factors. For instance, to cope up with the pains of imprisonment, the inmate becomes prisonized and adheres to inmate code; one of the codes may be homosexuality and drug-related behaviour. Moreover, the behaviour of prison inmates living with HIV may also be influenced by their evaluation of the 'staff world'.

The following pages highlight the experiences of prison inmates living with HIV in terms of prison living conditions, risk behaviour during incarceration, prison medical facilities, and adherence to ethical issues.

© The Author(s) 2015
S. Guin, *Prison Inmates Living with HIV in India*,
SpringerBriefs in Criminology, DOI 10.1007/978-3-319-15566-1_4

Prison Living Condition

Overcrowding

Four inmates referred space crunch as the major problem in one of the prisons. One of them was languishing as an undertrial and the rest of the three were referred for ART treatment. J. J. Hospital in Mumbai is the referral centre for treatment from all over Maharashtra. Prisoners from all over Maharashtra are referred to the prison in Mumbai for treatment at J. J. Hospital. This was one of the major causes of overcrowding. Three inmates were arrested under the Narcotic Drugs and Psychotropic Substances Act 1985 Act. As stated by UNAIDS (2004), the Prohibitionist policies against illicit drugs are fuelling overcrowding and HIV epidemic in prisons.

In one of the prisons, inmates were crammed together. As observed by the researcher and as mentioned by the doctor of the prison hospital, patients with HIV-related illness were put in the emergency ward, which was inside the hospital circle. In this ward, people who were sick and had ailments like Tuberculosis (TB), asthma, and other diseases were put together. Overcrowding was mostly due to the large number of undertrials, which accounted for more than 96 % of the inmates.

According to the ***prison staff*** of the prisons in Nasik and Pune, the living condition inside these two prisons was far better than that of the prison in Mumbai, which was overcrowded. The prison staff of the prison in Mumbai were of the same opinion. In a capacity of 804 inmates, the prison in Mumbai had an average of 3,000 prisoners. The Superintendent of the prison lamented on the situation of overcrowding, '...*we cannot stretch the living space...!*'

Data (NCRB 2012) reveal that as on 31st December 2013, the total number of prisoners in 1,394 prisons in the country was 385,135, with a total sanctioned strength of 343,169. Although the occupancy rate was 99.4 % in Maharashtra prisons (NCRB 2012), overcrowding was reported in Mumbai, Pune, and Nasik prisons, with occupancy rates being 363.06 %, 164.70 %, and 112.70 %, respectively (Raghavan and Nair 2011). The total sanctioned capacity in Yerwada Central Jail, Mumbai Central Jail, and Nasik Road Central Jail was 2,449, 804, and 3,178, respectively, and the actual capacity in these jails was 3,378, 2,162, and 2,151, respectively (NCRB 2012). Thus, Yerwada and Mumbai Central Jails were overcrowded. The situation of overcrowding in jails is aptly described by Bedi (2002) to be 'virtually bursting at the seams'.

Inmates of two of the three prisons reported that there was no problem of sanitation, hygiene, and drinking water. However, overcrowding had a serious impact on sanitation and hygiene in the other prison. Water supplied by the respective municipal corporations was used for both drinking and cleaning purposes. Since the supply was only for a limited period during the day, it was stored in tankers.

It emerges from the above that health condition of an inmate living with HIV may deteriorate in overcrowded spaces where inmates having multiple diseases are put together. It can impede efforts to deal with HIV and AIDS. It can worsen the health problems of those who are already ill and may also lead to increased high-risk behaviours. Overcrowding generates stress and boredom due to reduced work and programme activities. The deplorable living conditions in prisons are also marked by stuffy and suffocating prison cells, lack of fresh air and sunlight, and hygiene (Madhurima 2009). These conditions are imperative to the health of prison inmates living with HIV.

Conditions of overcrowding in prisons are also linked to the spread of TB. TB is an airborne communicable disease which spreads easily in crammed places with poor sanitary conditions. Thus, it may be said that overcrowding has a direct bearing on many aspects of a prisoner's life including hygiene and care, leading to the deterioration of health conditions.

Food and Nutrition

One of the most common complaints raised by all the seven inmates was about the quality of food. Although all inmates living with HIV were receiving special medical diet, every one of them complained of the poor and substandard quality of food, which was not conducive to their digestive system. Food was served thrice a day. The menu of the lunch and dinner was almost similar and consisted of rice, daal (lentils), one vegetable curry, and three to four chapattis (handmade wheat bread). Although milk was served as part of the special diet, it was mostly adulterated with water. The food was uncooked and spicy in nature. One inmate complained that he was not provided with any kind of protein, neither in the form of medicine nor through protein-rich diet. He felt that proper nutritious food was the only treatment for HIV patients to help them stay healthy. Another inmate, who was unable to eat the prison food, could manage to get permission for having home-cooked food, as he was an undertrial inmate. One of the inmates mentioned the difference in the special medical diet in the two prisons where he had stayed. He stated that the food in the prison where he was initially lodged was better. Supporting his views, he explained that as part of the special diet, he used to get two eggs, milk, one piece of bread, one apple, and two bananas, whereas in prison where he was lodged at the time of interview, special diet consisted only of bread, banana, and milk, and the allocation of eggs along with this special diet was meant only for the TB patients. Moreover, two inmates complained of **corruption** inside the prisons where money seemed to have played a role in getting better food, bigger space, and better treatment inside the prison. An inmate pointed out:

> If one wants to have good food and has money, he just needs to intimate this to the warder[1] of that particular barrack and the message is passed on to the prison guard. The prison guard

---

[1]Convicted long-term prisoners are appointed as prison warders based on certain criteria (Maharashtra Prison Manual 1979).

then manages to get better food for the inmate in lieu of an amount between Rs. 300 and 400. This food has special daal with tadka (tempering) and special chapatti (handmade wheat bread), which are of good quality and palatable. One can get anything in exchange of money.

It emerges from the above that although egg, milk, banana, apples, and bread are added as part of the special diet meant for inmates living with HIV, food remained a major concern for all the seven inmates. Consuming milk, banana, and bread as special diet wouldn't help if the main course of food is unpalatable. Although majority of budget (60.6 %) allocated for prison inmates was spent on food (NCRB 2012), food has remained one of the major issues for complaints by the prisoners. Inmates have complained of insect-infected wheat (Saini 2008) and adulterated milk (Bedi 2002).

It has been noted that poor nutritional status may hasten progression to AIDS-related illnesses (Gillespie 2005) and good nutrition is essential for keeping people living with HIV healthy. Moreover, nutritional diet enables them to resist opportunistic infections such as TB for long (UNAIDS n.d.). Thus, poor quality of food and improper nutrition may have a negative impact on the health of inmates living with HIV as proper nutrition and vitamins may postpone the development of HIV into AIDS (Goyer 2003).

Stress

All seven inmates highlighted that there was no one from outside the prison with whom they could discuss about the disease. As one inmate pointed out,

> If I want to discuss anything related to the disease, I talk to my friends. So far, I have not seen anyone to come here and talk about the disease. It's only you…"

Another inmate shared that he came to know about HIV and AIDS from fellow inmates (and later the doctor in the Government hospital) who told him about the symptoms of HIV and AIDS and modes of transmission. Four inmates shared their woes with other inmates who were living with HIV. One inmate commented that even the slightest discomfort in the body troubled him as his mind was always preoccupied about the disease. Another inmate requested the researcher to facilitate his transfer to a prison in West Bengal so that his family could meet him on a regular basis. This clearly indicates the need of emotional and psychological support, which is absent within the prison.

It emerges from the above that stress is an important area of concern as there is no support system available inside the prisons for stress-related issues of inmates living with HIV and AIDS. It may be mentioned that being imprisoned in itself carries with it a lot of stress, as a result of separation from the family and other support structures, frustration of goals or plans for the future, and interruption of family activities. This heavy psychological burden of imprisonment is intensified when the prisoner comes to know that he is HIV positive. Further in the absence of any support system available within the prison, the prison inmate living with HIV may become highly stressed, leading to a significant negative impact on his health. There is a need to include emotional and psychological support system as an integral part of providing care for an HIV-positive prisoner's health and well-being (Goyer 2003).

Risk Behaviour During Incarceration Inside Prisons

All seven inmates agreed to the fact that they had 'heard' about the occurrence of homosexuality inside prisons and gave their own estimate of the approximate prevalence rates of homosexuality. The views of prison inmates regarding homosexuality in prison appear to be contradictory. Some undertrial prisoners in Focus Group Discussions mentioned that incidents of homosexuality were possible only in prisons where long-term convicts were incarcerated. One inmate added that homosexuality was not possible in prisons due to the overcrowding. In contrary to this view, the focus group discussion with the other prisoners in the other two jails revealed that homosexuality was mainly possible in prisons where most inmates were undertrials. The latter view is in congruence with a study conducted in Mumbai Central Prison (Palve et al. 2006) where 72 % of a sample of 752 (75 employees and 677 inmates) said that they thought sex between men was common in prisons and 11 % were engaged in homosexual activities inside the prison. The prison staff across three prisons negated the existence of homosexuality. This may be because of the fact that homosexuality is an offence in India (Mahapatra 2013) and its occurrence in the prison premises would mean the inefficiency of the prison administration in maintaining discipline. The views of prison medical doctors regarding the prevalence of homosexuality were similar to the other prison staff. Only the medical doctor at one of the prisons felt that the prevalence of homosexuality could be roughly around 5–10 %, although he pointed out that he never came across any such cases since his joining the prison hospital. Sex between inmates was reported in women prison and in male prison (Donde 2006; Bedi 2002).

Studies indicate that prison inmates engage in homosexuality due to several factors like 'frustration', 'long accumulations of sexual energy', 'submission out of fear', or 'submission in return for protection or other favours' (Burstein 1977). Goyer (2003) notes that distributing condoms and lubricants is advocated by the World Health Organization and UNAIDS. However, homosexuality being an offence in many countries, it is difficult to get authorities to acknowledge homosexual activity inside the prison. This prevents the development of condom policies in some countries. Thus, prison population is at risk of getting infected with HIV through sexual transmission.

As a follow-up of the National Training Programme to address HIV prevention amongst incarcerated substance users, UNODC and Sankalp (an NGO in Mumbai) organized a one-day sensitization programme on HIV and AIDS inside the prison in Mumbai premises for the inmates and staff including the prison personnel, prison medical doctor, and paramedical staff. In this sensitization programme, the inmates participated in the various events conducted by Sankalp and even performed a skit depicting the various ways through which HIV may get transmitted to inmates inside the prisons. The skit highlighted homosexuality in exchange for better sleeping space and drugs, and how poor inmates gave in to the demands to receive monetary and other favours.

Homosexuality is prohibited under Section 377 of the Indian Penal Code, 1860,[2] and any activity abetting this behaviour is illegal.

While the senior prison officials believed providing condoms to be a contentious issue, it is essential to introduce condoms inside the prisons as homosexuality is a reality in prisons all over the world and India is no exception. Homosexuality is prevalent in the society, and prison is a part of the larger society. People who come to prisons may also have had homosexual encounters prior to incarceration either consensually or coerced. They may thus become involved in homosexual behaviours inside the prison with consent or without consent, which may in turn become a major cause of transmission of HIV.

Although there is no prevalence data regarding drug use and tattooing in Indian prisons (Dolan & Larney 2010), availability and access to alcohol and injectable or oral drugs such as heroin and marijuana were reported inside prison and needles and syringes were reused and shared (Chakrapani et al. 2013). Interpersonal violence between prisoners leading to lacerations, bites, and bleeding was reported from a Mumbai prison presenting the risk of HIV transmission (Donde 2006).

Health Delivery System Inside the Prison

Three inmates highlighted the faulty medical treatment methods in the prison. According to them, they contracted HIV due to the negligence of the medical staff in the prison who used non-sterilized needles. However, two of the three inmates agreed that they contracted HIV in the 1990s when knowledge and awareness regarding HIV was less and the use of disposable syringes was not common. The third inmate blamed it on the negligence of the prison staff.

Prison inmates living with HIV were referred to the Government hospital only when their health condition deteriorated. There was no treatment available for prison inmates living with AIDS inside the prison. Even for simple blood tests and other check-ups, inmates had to be referred to the Government hospital. The prison staff also mentioned that there was no adequate specialized medical service available inside the prison and only the instrument for checking blood pressure was available.

---

[2] Indian Penal Code, 1860, is a document which lists offences and punishments that a person committing any crime is charged with.

The *prison doctors and the prison staff* explained the procedure for receiving medical treatment inside the prisons. If an inmate felt sick and wanted to meet the doctor, he informed the circle warder. The inmate could also inform the jailor during his rounds from morning 8 a.m. to 12 p.m. and in the afternoon from 4 p.m. to 6 p.m. The circle jailor allowed such inmates to meet the doctor at the hospital OPD. Inmates could also meet the doctor directly during his visits in the particular circle. The Medical Officer (MO) diagnosed them and prescribed medicines. If there was any need to isolate them or admit them, the MO admitted them in the prison hospital ward. If required, such inmates were sent to the Government Hospital for further treatment. Inmates were referred to Government hospital when they did not respond to the treatment provided at the prison hospital or had serious health condition or due to lack of equipment for conducting pathological tests (like blood and serum testing, etc.). The patients who were seriously ill were referred to the Government Hospital (i.e. J. J. Hospital in Mumbai, Sassoon Hospital in Pune, and Nasik Government Hospital in Nasik). The doctors at the Government hospital decided the course of treatment for the particular prisoner.

There was no medical examination of any prisoner during admission[3] in the prison regardless of whether he was an undertrial or a convict. During admission, the inmates were only asked about their identification mark, and the height and weight were noted. The doctors and the prison staff agreed that inmates were attended to only when they complained of their health situation. Before admission to the prison, inmates were taken to the Government hospital and were asked if they had any physical problems. Here, most of them were found to be suffering from skin diseases, upper respiratory tract infections like cough and cold, and other ailments like hypertension, diabetes, etc. The prison doctors also supplemented that during admission in the prison, prisoners were asked about their identification mark and their height and weight were measured and noted. One of the CMOs shared the fact that sometimes prisoners faked illness, as they wanted to get out of prison to the Government hospital. As a result, the CMO had to identify the genuine cases. Sometimes prisoners tried to convince the CMO to get themselves referred to the Government hospital. In such situations, the CMO referred only those patients who were seriously ill and needed to be referred to the Government hospital for further treatment.

One inmate living with HIV mentioned that for minor ailments like indigestion, they were provided medicines available in the prison hospital, which were ineffective.

---

[3] According to the Maharashtra Prison Manual 1979, inmates have to be subjected to preliminary physical examination to check whether the prisoner is suffering from any contagious disease. The NHRC guidelines require that all State Governments and prison administrations should ensure medical examination of all the prison inmates prior to admission in accordance with the proforma devised by it and the monthly reports be communicated to the Commission.

According to the prison staff, general medical care and preliminary treatment for inmates were available inside the prison. They explained:

Doctors were available round the clock. There was a prison hospital as specified in the Prison Manual. The prison doctor attended to medical complaints of the inmates and provided primary treatment including medicine, which were available inside the prison. Medicines which were not available inside the prison were bought from outside whenever needed. Budget was available to buy required medicines. The doctor had the discretion to decide if someone had to be admitted in the prison hospital. Inmates living with HIV developed opportunistic infections like TB or skin disease. The prison doctor provided primary treatment which was available inside the prison. If the inmate didn't respond to treatment inside the prison or if he required further specialized treatment, the doctor referred the inmate for further treatment to the Government hospital. Sometimes, even for simple medical requirements like conducting an X-ray, the inmate had to be referred to the Government Hospital. The Superintendent had to arrange for police escort for the same. All three Government hospitals were equipped with Voluntary Counseling and Testing Centres (VCTC) where blood test for HIV was conducted. In Mumbai, J. J. Hospital had the Antiretroviral Therapy (ART) Centre, which provided the treatment for inmate living with HIV, based on the inmate's CD4 count. All inmates living with HIV inside the Mumbai Central Prison were registered with the Antiretroviral Therapy Centre at the J. J. Hospital. This Centre provided ART free of cost. In Pune, ART was available in the Sassoon Hospital where the inmates were referred to from the Yerwada Central Jail. However, in Nasik, the Government hospital didn't have ART centre, so the inmates requiring further treatment for HIV were referred to the J. J. Hospital in Mumbai, by the doctor in the Nasik Government hospital. Inmates suffering from TB underwent the DOTS treatment, through the respective Government hospitals.

As observed by the researcher and according to the prison doctors, one of the prisons had a two-storied hospital without facilities such as an X-ray or ECG machine to examine a patient at the time of an emergency. Even the stock of medicines at the hospital was limited to first-aid items and drugs used for treatment of minor ailments. For any major HIV-related illness, the prisoners were entirely dependent on J. J. Hospital or their own family members for medicines. A higher prison official retorted that undertrials from all over Maharashtra were referred to the government hospital in Mumbai for better treatment and thus were lodged in the prison in Mumbai. One inmate shared that due to the problem of non-availability of guard escorts, sick inmates were taken to the Government hospital only when their condition became critical.

All seven prisoners reported non-availability of police escort when referred to Government hospital. Even when the guard was provided, they used to reach Government hospital after the scheduled timing of the OPD. Prison staff explained that it was due to the lack of manpower and non-availability of cars to escort the inmates. This situation delayed treatment, and sometimes treatment was discontinued for a prolonged period. A respondent in the Focus Group Discussion shared that prisoners had to be escorted to the Government hospital by a minimum of two police guards. Thus, treatment of inmates living with HIV became a long-drawn-out process as non-availability of police escorts resulted in delay and discontinuation of treatment.

Treatment for HIV-Related Diseases

Four inmates suffered from TB as the major opportunistic infection and got cured through DOTS. Tuberculosis is one of the most common opportunistic infections for people living with HIV, which poses a substantial danger to their health condition by accelerating the progress of AIDS (Lines & Stover 2005). HIV infection is the most potent risk factor to convert latent TB into active transmissible TB. TB has been identified as one of the leading causes of death among HIV-positive individuals internationally. Moreover, many prisoners who might have been detected HIV positive inside the prison, after a secondary infection like TB, could actually have got infected outside the prison (UNAIDS 1997).

Thus, the conditions of overcrowding, poor nutrition, impediments in accessing continued medical care, high turnover of population, poor health education, and high-risk behaviour in the prison present a number of risk factors for HIV–TB co-infection.

The prison doctors and prison staff reiterated that all inmates living with HIV were receiving special medical diet. Whenever an inmate living with HIV fell sick, all the necessary steps were taken to ensure that the disease was cured without delay. However, the government hospital did not have the facility to test the CD4 count and did not have an ART centre. As a result, an inmate had to be referred to the referral hospital at Mumbai for the CD4 count, and thereafter the patient had to be sent for treatment every 6 months. According to the CMO of one of the prisons, the medical facilities available for people living with HIV and AIDS inside the prison was better than that available in the community. He explained that in prison, the inmate was getting treatment and medicines free of cost apart from the food, which the inmate might not get if he was out in the community. However, the view of the prisoners on this was exactly the opposite. They stressed on the need for an improvement in the basic facilities like food and medical treatment.

It is evident from the above that there was no particular treatment facility available to the inmates living with AIDS. No special measures were taken to ensure that the inmates living with AIDS were provided with the most appropriate treatment available either within the prison or in the referral centres (Government Hospitals).

There were Voluntary Counseling and Testing Centres (VCTC) at the Government Hospitals where the blood could be tested for HIV and pre- and post-test counseling was provided. Although the ART was available in Mumbai and Pune (J. J. Hospital and Sassoon Hospital, respectively), the HIV-positive inmates of Nasik jail faced huge problem in accessing ART due to the cumbersome referral procedure and non-availability of guard escorts. Although all inmates living with HIV were provided with special medical diet consisting mostly of milk and bread, the quality of the food provided was substandard and inadequate for people living with HIV.

Ethical Issues

Testing

There was no facility inside the prison for HIV testing. When an inmate was diagnosed with an opportunistic infection, like TB or lung infection, and didn't respond to treatment in the prison hospital, he was referred for further treatment at the Government Hospital. It was the doctor at the Government hospital who decided whether the patient should go for an HIV testing or not. It was only when the doctor suggested the inmate to go for the test that the HIV status of the patient was determined.

Prior to HIV testing, informed consent was taken from four inmates, who also received pre- and post-test counseling. Apprehensive of his own health condition, because of the prolonged illness, one of the inmates requested the prison doctor to help him get his blood tested for HIV. In case of two inmates, informed consent was not taken for HIV testing. Moreover, neither of them received pre- and post-test counselling. The inmate who himself had requested for HIV testing was not informed of his test results by the doctor. He came to know that he was HIV positive from a fellow prisoner only when he insisted on the report. The doctor at the Government hospital communicated the test results to four inmates. In case of one inmate, the communication of test results was done by the prison doctor. One of the inmates was intimated his test result by one of the fellow prisoners who was working in the prison hospital as nursing orderly. According to the prison doctor at Mumbai Central Prison, every month the blood samples of around 10–15 prisoners were tested for HIV at the Voluntary Counselling and Testing Centre.

Confidentiality

Provision of special diet became an ethical issue, as prisoners who were receiving special diet were easily identified by other prisoners. This was an issue for three prison inmates living with HIV. In one of the prisons, it was observed by the researcher that 'HIV positive' was written on the medical files of the inmates living with HIV (the researcher had to obtain special permission from the IG prisons in order to get access to the medical and other records of the respective inmates, on conditions of confidentiality). Thus, the nursing orderlies who worked in the prison hospital and the police guards who escorted the inmates living with HIV and handled the medical records could easily identify inmates living with HIV. Three inmates were ready to disclose their HIV-positive status if such disclosure helped them in receiving better medical treatment or other benefits. For example, one inmate wanted to get transferred to a prison in his home state, West Bengal, and had officially requested to take his health condition into consideration, for the same. Another inmate who had requested that his health condition required proper quality diet, which was not provided inside the prison, was permitted to have home-cooked food.

Discrimination

Incidents of discrimination against prison inmates living with HIV, on the grounds of their HIV-positive status, were not reported by any of the respondents. Inmates living with HIV were allowed to work if they were physically capable and wanted to work. They had access to other places like kitchen. Six inmates shared that the behaviour of the police guards and the medical doctors was not proper; they were either rude or didn't talk to them amiably, though this was not because of their HIV-positive status but simply because of the fact that they were prisoners. However, one inmate shared an incident where the attitude of the police guard (who was escorting him to the Government hospital) towards him changed as soon as the inmate informed the guard that he was HIV positive. Two inmates specifically pointed out the inappropriate behaviour of the doctors at one Government hospital, but they felt that this was basically because they were prisoners and had nothing to do with their HIV-positive status.

Segregation

Only one inmate shared that he was kept in a separate single cell in one prison when he was detected with HIV as the prison doctor felt that the skin disease he was suffering from might spread to other inmates. However, it was unclear if the skin disease was contagious. Other prison inmates living with HIV were never asked to stay in separate cells. It was the prison doctor who decided whether an inmate needed to be kept separate in cases where the inmate had a contagious disease like TB. The CMO of one prison was aware of the World Health Organization (WHO) guidelines on HIV infection and AIDS in prison (UNAIDS 1999). According to the WHO guidelines, segregating prison inmates living with HIV only on the grounds of their HIV-positive status is an offence. Prisoners living with HIV having secondary infection and suffering from a communicable disease like TB were kept separate because of the contagious nature of the disease. The Superintendent of one prison shared that people living with HIV should be kept separate in order to avoid any kind of harassment from those who were not HIV positive.

> If the inmates living with HIV are kept in the same barrack with others, then those who are not HIV positive may harass them. Other inmates may not treat the HIV positive prisoners with the basic dignity and respect because being HIV positive carries a lot of stigma. They may not speak with them properly, nor eat or talk to them. This may lead to inferiority complex. There

is a need to spread the right kind of message regarding HIV and AIDS, because many inmates still carry a lot of misconception and misinformation about HIV and AIDS.

It is clear from the above that maintaining confidentiality is an issue in the prison. The medical reports of the patients were kept in the custody of the prison doctor, ensuring confidentiality from the doctors' side. These were supposed to be confidential reports, available only to the patient, the medical doctor, and the superintendent of the prison (if required). However, people assisting the medical doctor like the nursing orderlies in the prison hospital were aware of the identity of the inmates living with HIV. This was because the HIV status of the inmate was written on top of the medical file (in one of the prison). Moreover, the guards who escorted the inmate to the Government hospital carried the medical files and thus the HIV-positive status of the respective prison inmate got revealed to them.

Preventive Measures Inside Prison

Only one inmate mentioned about an NGO, representatives of which were occasionally visiting the prison to provide counselling to the inmates living with HIV. This fact was supported by the prison doctors and other staff. Three inmates shared that they got information regarding HIV and AIDS from TV and newspapers; one of them even collected newspaper cuttings related to HIV. Two inmates mentioned about posters on HIV which were on display in the prison hospital premises. One inmate shared that once a video show on HIV was organized in the prison. According to the prison doctor and prison staff, various organizations conducted programmes inside the prison which included recreational events, health camps, eye camps, and legal aid. In one prison, the District AIDS Control Society had circulated pamphlets on HIV and AIDS and conducted voluntary counselling. In another prison, non-governmental organizations occasionally visited the prison to conduct *satsangs* (spiritual prayers), musical events, orchestra, etc., but none of them were working on HIV and AIDS. The Superintendent of one prison shared the sporadic visits made by NGOs in the following words:

> NGOs are required only for counseling and giving lectures on HIV and AIDS. NGOs cannot provide continued treatment of AIDS, as they are irregular. Only the Government agency can conduct testing of HIV. If the treatment of AIDS is not regular, it affects the CD 4 count of the person living with HIV.

In Mumbai, there were different NGOs working on various health-related issues. The NGO by the name Sankalp was specifically working on drug de-addiction and sometimes visited the prison to provide counselling to the HIV-positive inmates. The Superintendent of one of the prisons felt that there was a need for NGOs to visit the prison and work on HIV and AIDS, especially on counseling, testing, and treatment. In Nasik there was not a single NGO which was working specifically on HIV and AIDS.

Conclusion

The analysis of the experiences of the prison inmates living with HIV reveals that two of the three central prisons were overcrowded. Food remained a major concern for all the seven inmates. Discussion revealed that there was an absence of emotional and psychological support system in the prison. Prison inmates concurred to the prevalence of homosexuality in jail. There was no treatment available for prison inmates living with AIDS. Non-availability of police escort was cited as the major problem faced by the prison inmate living with HIV which hampered continuity of care and treatment. It is evident that ethical issues regarding confidentiality were violated. However, no discrimination on the grounds of HIV-positive status was indicated by the prison inmates living with HIV.

Chapter 5
Prison Personnel and HIV: Views and Experiences

In order to achieve a holistic picture of the situation of HIV inside the prisons, it is essential that along with the experiences of prison inmates living with HIV, the views and experiences of the prison medical team and the prison staff are also taken into account.

This chapter presents the views of the prison medical team and the prison staff regarding the situation of HIV and AIDS in prisons. The data were gathered through an unstructured interview with the prison doctors and staff and are presented under various subthemes.

Structure of Prison Hospital and Hospital Staff

The data gathered from the medical doctors in the prison regarding the structure of prison hospital and working pattern of the hospital staff are presented below.

Mumbai Central Jail

This prison had five wards in the prison hospital, namely the in-patient ward or the general ward, the tuberculosis ward, the emergency ward, the minor ailment ward, and the infectious disease ward.

Apart from the Chief Medical Officer (CMO), there were three doctors and two pharmacists. Four nursing orderlies from the prison staff had first aid training and worked as helper as well as security men.

The CMO was responsible both for administrative and supervisory work. He attended to the health-related issues of prison inmates and was also engaged in court-related matters. Court-related matters consisted of helping prisoners with their

© The Author(s) 2015
S. Guin, *Prison Inmates Living with HIV in India*,
SpringerBriefs in Criminology, DOI 10.1007/978-3-319-15566-1_5

health-related issues and getting bail on medical grounds. Sometimes, the court also directed the CMO to send his report regarding a particular prisoner. One of the medical officers looked after the daily OPD (Out Patient Department) and conducted health check-up of newly admitted prison inmates. The other medical officer served night duty working from 8 p.m. to 8 a.m. and spent the night in the prison.

Yerwada Central Jail

The Yerwada Central Jail hospital had five wards—the general ward (with 25 beds), the TB ward with 20 beds, the leprosy ward with 10–15 beds, a separate ward for patients with contagious/communicable diseases like cholera and hepatitis, which was also used for psychiatric patients (20 beds), and the *Buddha* (aged) ward meant for inmates above the age of 60. On average, there were 42–50 old inmates.

Apart from the Chief Medical Officer, there was a psychiatrist who looked after the psychiatric patients. There were two Medical Officers who were in charge of all administrative and office work. Another two Medical Officers looked after all clinical work and the OPD. There was one psychologist and six nursing orderlies. One pharmacist looked after the medical store. There were two compounders who were mostly engaged in dispensing medicines in the OPD and keeping record regarding medical diet.

Nasik Road Central Jail

The prison hospital consisted of four wards, namely the general ward, the psychiatric ward, the tuberculosis ward, and the Geriatric ward. More than sixty patients on an average were admitted in the prison hospital. The medical staff consisted of a Chief Medical Officer and a Medical Officer. Two pharmacists were appointed by the prison. There were four nursing orderlies who had undergone a training of 3 months on first aid. Apart from these personnel, there was a psychiatrist who visited the prison once or twice a week.

Working Pattern of the Medical Staff

In Mumbai Central Jail, the OPD was functional from 9 a.m. to 12 p.m. and from 4 p.m. to 5 p.m. General physical examination of about 200–300 prisoners was conducted on a daily basis. On an average, around 10–15 prisoners were diagnosed every day as seriously ill, who needed referral to the government hospital. Serious illness included fever not responding to treatment at the prison hospital. The doctors attended to emergency calls. After 6 p.m., the prisoners were locked inside barracks. Doctors were available on call 24 hours within the prison premise.

In Yerwada Central Jail, the first shift of OPD was from 8 a.m. to 2 p.m. during which one medical officer took rounds of each circle accompanied by the compounder and the nursing orderly. In each circle, the doctor examined patients complaining of minor ailments. Thereafter, the doctor started the OPD. In Nasik Road Central Jail, the OPD started at 10.30 a.m. and continued till 1.30 p.m. and resumed from 4.30 p.m. to 6 p.m.

Appointment

All doctors were appointed by the Directorate of Health Services, Government of Maharashtra. They were deputed for one year from the Directorate of Health Service to the Department of Prison.

The prison medical service in most states in India is in the dual control of the prison department and the Directorate of Medical and Health Services (DMHS). Appointments are made by the DMHS and the prison department has no authority to recruit medical officers based on specific health needs of prison inmates. Generally, one deputy surgeon, one assistant surgeon, and one pathologist are appointed at each central prison and one assistant surgeon is appointed for each district jail. According to the prison authorities, the reason for appointment of doctors on deputation instead of direct recruitment is that posting in prison is not considered as a prospective avenue for a career (Karnam 2009).

Training Before Deputation in Prison

Before being appointed as prison doctors, the medical officers did not undergo any training regarding the prison structure and systems.

Karnam (2009) notes the lack of specific policy guidelines on the appointment of prison medical personnel addressing the needs of the prison population.

HIV in Prisons

The Chief Medical Officer of one prison shared the following view regarding HIV infection among inmates:

> …presence of HIV in the blood causes immune suppression. This means that a person living with HIV will have a weak immune system and will be prone to other opportunistic infections like TB, skin diseases etc. Prisoners are usually hesitant to go for HIV test, as

most of them are aware of their high risk behavior and sexual history and don't want to reveal it. It is only when they suffer from other diseases and the health condition deteriorates that they go for the HIV test voluntarily or are referred for the test and are detected with HIV. In the mean time, there is a huge time gap between the time of infection and detection of the HIV and the virus gets sufficient time to weaken the immune system of the patient. During admission to the jail, the prisoner is asked about his medical history, if he has any sexually transmitted disease and, whether he was involved in any high risk behavior, but most of the prisoners do not reveal this information until they are severely ill.

The Chief Medical Officer of another prison shared his opinion about how the inmates got infected with HIV:

HIV is diagnosed based on the signs and syndromes of the disease and the clinical history plays a pivotal role in HIV infection. If the inmate has had multiple unsafe sexual contacts, he is most likely to contract the virus. There is no way that HIV may spread inside the prison. If there is any history of blood transfusion of the inmate while he was outside the prison or if he has a history of homosexuality outside the prison, then the person is more likely to carry the virus inside prison. There are no cases of Injecting Drug Abuse inside the prison. Moreover, there are no prisoners who are addicts as no one suffers from withdrawal symptoms. There have been no complains where it might be inferred that two men might have indulged in sex. This is because there have been no cases so far where any inmate has complained of bleeding from the anal region, which could be an outcome of homosexual act. However, the rate of homosexuality in the prison might be 5–10 %. The usual symptoms of HIV are opportunistic infections and drastic weight loss. Hence, it is easy to detect HIV. If a person contracts HIV and is subjected to ELISA test within the first 3 months of infection, the test result may be negative. This period of 3 months is called the "window period". Many inmates are aware of HIV and AIDS. There may be 5 % inmates who are ignorant about the disease.

The CMO of another jail felt that all inmates living with HIV got infected when they were outside the prison. He negated the occurrence of homosexuality inside the prison and thus the spread of the HIV through homosexuality within the prison.

Liaison with the Prison Staff

There was no interference of the prison authorities in the work of the prison doctors. Instead the prison staff offered friendly support and provided necessary cooperation whenever required. However, it was observed by the researcher during her visits that the prison doctors were quite apprehensive to answer the questions of the researcher. There had been several occasions when the doctors were reluctant to share facts regarding the prisoners. The researcher had to acquire a separate permission from the Inspector General of Prisons, Maharashtra, to access the medical and other records (to go through the medical files) of the inmates living with HIV, in spite of the fact that she already had permission to undertake the research.

Problems Faced by Prison Doctors

Lack of Lab Technician

The post of the Lab Technician was vacant for a long time. The preceding Lab Technician, just after joining, had requested for various lab equipments from the Inspector General of Prisons, Maharashtra. However, the technician resigned from the job and left. Presence of a lab technician helped the doctors in minor medical investigations within the prison, without having to refer the inmate to the Government Hospital. Minor investigations included simple blood tests, haemoglobin test, test of white blood cells and red blood cells, blood sugar, urine test, etc.

Insufficient Number of Prison Medical Doctors

One of the prisons was established in the year 1871 with a capacity of 2,323 inmates. One day, it was recorded that there were 3,734 inmates within that prison. The number of doctors and equipments in the prison did not increase keeping pace with the increase in the number of inmates. The number of inmates was too many for the few prison doctors to handle. There was requirement of more medical officers due to overcrowding of prisons.

Inadequate Equipments and Medical Supplies Within the Prison

Only preliminary treatment was available in the prison for the inmates. The prison hospital did not have the basic equipments for medical investigation like blood test, X-ray machine, etc. The medical supplies in the prison hospital are limited to bare minimum medicines, equivalent almost to a first aid centre.

Suggestions Offered by the Prison Doctors

Testing

According to the CMO of one of the prisons, doctors from Government hospital should visit the prison to conduct the ELISA test.

Another CMO remarked,

> HIV testing should be made mandatory at the initial stage during the medical checkup of an accused/ convict when he/she is transferred from the police custody to the judicial custody. Usually, when an accused/convict is sent to the judicial custody from the police custody, it

is mandatory according to the Prison Manual to send him for medical checkup. During this check up, it should be made mandatory that the prisoner undergoes HIV test through the spot/ card test. If this is done at this stage itself, then precautions can be taken for the inmate who is tested HIV positive and his/her treatment can be started immediately, if required. Also, such prisoner can be protected from contracting other contagious diseases like TB inside the prison. Moreover, if the HIV screening test was conducted within the prison premises, most of the prisoners would come forward and voluntarily go for HIV test.

Homosexual Activity

A medical officer of one prison acknowledged the occurrence of homosexuality in that prison in the following words:

There should be a check on homosexual activities inside the prison. It should be a concern for the prison authorities to take steps in this regard.

Involvement of NGOs

Many inmates who did not have any history of unsafe sexual behaviour had requested the CMO of the prison to arrange for HIV testing. However, as there was no such facility available in the prison, the voluntary testing could not be conducted. Hence, if a Non-Governmental Organization, in collaboration with the prison authorities, organized HIV counselling and testing inside the prison, there would be scope for early detection of HIV. Requirement for Voluntary Counselling and Testing Centre was felt inside the prison for HIV counselling and testing.

One doctor remarked,

Presently, NGOs working in prison are not undertaking any treatment or rehabilitation programmes for inmates suffering from HIV and AIDS. Such NGOs should be given permission to work with the prison administration so that they can help the HIV positive inmates with treatment and rehabilitation. The NGO Sankalp has a Drop in Centre. Sankalp can get the prisoners who are being released, registered with this Centre and work on their treatment and follow up.

Pre-release

The necessity of pre-release of inmates living with HIV was voiced by one doctor in a prison.

Pre release or early release should be encouraged. On the recommendation of the prison CMO, the Superintendent of the prison could send a pre-release proposal to the Government and the Government should then consider the pre-release of the inmates living with HIV & AIDS.

Medical Care in Prisons

The opinion of medical doctors regarding medical care in prison clearly indicates limited resources for medical care inside prison.

> The medical facilities available in the prison are bare minimum. There has to be a laboratory inside the prison for minor pathological tests (e.g. Urine test). Basic equipments like ECG machine, X-Ray Machine and more number of oxygen cylinders are required. Many a times, an inmate has to be sent to the JJ Hospital for minor tests. Most often, there is a problem of availability of guard to escort the inmate to the Hospital. If a laboratory is set up inside the prison, the prison doctors themselves can carry out the tests and go ahead with the subsequent treatment based on the test results. This will minimize the problem of guard allotment to escort inmates to the hospital. Specialist doctors should visit the prison and treat inmates in the premises for skin infections, sexually transmitted diseases etc.

> A well-equipped sub district level civil hospital was required inside the prison. Such hospitals have facilities of X-Ray and operation theatre. If such provisions were made inside the prison premises, then inmates would not be required to be referred to the city hospital thus reducing the problem of guard allotment.

Overcrowding

The medical staff mentioned the problem of overcrowding in prisons hampering effective medical care in prison and making inmates vulnerable to several diseases.

> Although around 400 low cost latrines are being constructed in the prison, overcrowding in the prison will still make the situation worse. There is ventilation and space problem. Overcrowding also makes inmates prone to the communicable diseases.

Prison Staff

Discussion with the Superintendents and Jailors of each of the three prisons led to the following revelations:

Ratio of Prison Staff to Inmates

In *Yerwada Central Prison*, there were 402 guarding staff available with the prison and there were 3,653 prisoners as on March 29, 2006. The staff worked in 3 shifts a day at three different sites—inside the prison, in the workshop, and in the vocational training centres. The average admission/release of prisoners per day was around 30–40.

As per the records of September 1st, 2006, of *Nasik Road Central Prison*, the number of prison inmates was 2,176 against the total capacity of 1,977 inmates.

In *Mumbai Central Prison*, the official data of September 1st, 2006 suggested that the number of inmates was 2,750 and that the number of staff was 200.

The cumulative data of the State of Maharashtra suggest that the prisons have a total staff strength of 50,358 jail officials to take care of 385,135 inmates, which amounts to one Jail Official per eight inmates. The highest ratio of number of inmates per prison staff was reported from Jharkhand (20), followed by Bihar (17), Chhattisgarh (15), Uttar Pradesh, and Uttarakhand (11 each), and Rajasthan and Gujarat (10 each) (NCRB 2012).

Thus, it is evident from the data that the number of staff compared to the number of prison inmates is very less. Mostly this is because of the problem of overcrowding. As a result, under these critical circumstances, it is quite stressful for the officials of the prison department to manage such a huge number of prisoners.

Reasons for HIV in Prisons

The staff of all the three prisons were of the opinion that prison inmates living with HIV got infected outside the prison. There was no way that they could have contracted the virus after admission inside the prison. Prison staff didn't come across any case of homosexuality. They were of the opinion that there were some inmates who knew that they were HIV positive or suspected themselves to be HIV positive due to their high-risk behaviour (when they were outside prison) but were not ready to accept the fact that they might be HIV positive. Even if some people were aware of their HIV-positive status before admission in the prison, they never disclosed their HIV status mainly because of the fear of stigma and discrimination. One prison Superintendent exclaimed:

> These people will die of secondary disease but will never disclose of their possible HIV positive status…Inside the jail, mostly the inmates are dying a natural death. The other major cause of deaths is Tuberculosis. There is a possibility that the inmates dying of TB are HIV positive as well. There may be many such cases of HIV positive inmates but most of such cases are unknown.

Training of Prison Staff on HIV and AIDS

The Superintendents shared that the training they received before joining the department did not have any curricula on HIV and AIDS, mainly because the infection was not that widespread and very little was known about the issue at that point of time. Consequently, the topic was not relevant enough to be included in the curricula for the training of prison staff. However, time has changed and HIV and AIDS are one of the major global concerns. Still at present, there was no training on HIV and AIDS in the curricula that is being imparted to the new batch of people joining the Prison Department. One of the Superintendents felt that information related to HIV and AIDS should be incorporated in the training module of the Prison Training Curricula. This information may include knowledge related to care, treatment, prevention, and counselling of people living with HIV. The training period for the Guard (*Sipahi*) is 5 months and that of Superintendents and Jailors is 1 year.

There were no official programmes of the Prison Department disseminating information on HIV and AIDS for the staff inside any of the three prisons. In two of the three prisons, NGOs occasionally organized programmes on HIV and AIDS and only the staff present in the prison during the programme attended such programmes. The prison staff felt that information related to HIV was not very significant for the staff, as they were aware and conscious about the disease. The staff rather felt that information on HIV was more crucial for prison inmates. In Mumbai Central Prison, Sion Hospital[1] was running a project, in which training of trainers (three workshops) programme was conducted for prison employees on HIV and AIDS. There were no reported cases of HIV and AIDS among the prison staff.

Peer Educators

There was no peer education programme in any of the three prisons. The Superintendent of one of the prisons agreed that peer educators inside the prison would be a viable solution to spread the message regarding the various aspects of HIV and AIDS amongst the inmates. Inmates, who were HIV positive, and were willing to help others, may be suitable to educate other inmates inside the prison. However, the Superintendent then shared some of the practical problems related to this. He said that during his rounds and visits inside the various barracks in the prison, he had heard inmates using filthy language. Hence, he believed that the inmates did not have any control over their language and could utter whatever they wanted. Besides, discussion on HIV and AIDS would involve discussion on human sexual habits. This, he felt, might lead to utterance and discussion of words, which were sexually laden or had sexual innuendos. In such a scenario, the whole seriousness of the issue might get lost and the discussion might fully divert to issues related to sexual priorities. Moreover, since the peer educator would be someone amongst them and not someone from outside without a criminal record, some inmates might refuse to listen to the peer educator. They might try to talk some other irrelevant topic. He tried to explain this fact by giving the example of the change in behaviour of the inmates in the presence of the researcher inside the prison.

---

[1] Lokmanya Tilak Municipal General Hospital, locally known as 'Sion Hospital', is a municipal hospital situated in Sion, a suburb of Mumbai.

You being a lady have a different impact on the usage of words and body language of the prisoners… (In your presence) they try to use decent and polished words instead of using dirty and derogatory language. Compared to a peer educator, a counselor from outside will be more effective in spreading the message relating to HIV and AIDS. Instead of discussing HIV and AIDS, they may start discussing their previous profession or the crimes committed by them. They may start discussing how to plan a theft or how to commit a crime. It's better that a counselor from outside should visit the jail.

However, as shared by prison inmates, among the inmates there were others who discussed on decent topics without using any bad language. These inmates constituted a separate group interested on spiritual issues. These two groups of people usually were separate due to their entirely different nature of discussion topics. The two groups would rarely mix and match with each other and often did not accept each other.

It is evident from the above that the Superintendent is very enthusiastic with the concept of peer educators. He feels that peer educators might turn out to be great assets in spreading HIV and AIDS knowledge and education within the prison. However, there are some practical issues which need to be dealt with in order to make things work. Before involving them in the HIV and AIDS awareness generation within the prison, HIV-positive inmates willing to be peer educators need to be properly trained by professionals. Engagement of external counsellors is the other viable option, though the acceptance level in terms of sharing of personal sexual behaviours by the inmates to an outsider is debatable.

Pre-release

The Superintendent of one prison shared that there is a provision of premature release for terminally ill prisoners. Such cases are being referred to the Government for further action, '… *we cannot ask for pre-release to the Government. We can just refer the file regarding pre release to the I.G., Prisons, and after that it depends on the Government to decide on that*'.

Premature release of prisoners is a concession or privilege extended by the State and the prisoner cannot claim it as a matter of right. It is based on the reformation philosophy. Premature release is realized through the 'review of sentences' undertaken in accordance with the special enactments, rules, or orders formulated by the respective State Governments. The system differs from State to State based on the eligibility criteria of the person being considered for premature release, the composition of the Sentence Review Boards, and the guidelines governing the question of premature release, but more often than not it has been observed that this system is not being followed (Tiwari 2006).

Major Problems Faced by the Prison Administration

One of the major problems that all the three prisons face on a regular basis is non-availability of police guards as and when required. The problem of non-availability of police guards is a major hindrance in the regular accessibility of treatment for the inmates living with HIV. As revealed during discussion with the prison officials, guards are provided by the Police Department for the prisons. However, most often these police guards meant for the prison work are utilized for the police work.

Suggestions Offered by Prison Staff

(a) Facilities inside the prison: All facilities and equipments (like ECG), which are available in a Primary Health Centre, should be available in the prison. This is because there is always a problem of availability of police guard to escort an inmate to the civil hospital. A prison guard can escort only in emergency cases. Such facilities will reduce this problem.

(b) Medical treatment for AIDS in prison: As regards to the problem of treatment of AIDS in prisons, ART treatment should be made available inside the prison. Staff from the Government Hospital should come for Voluntary Testing and Counselling in the prison and provide counselling and necessary treatment within the prison.

(c) Involvement of NGOs: Some NGOs and community-based organizations should work on HIV and AIDS inside the prison regularly and consistently. Most of them come occasionally and mostly for their own publicity.

(d) Aftercare: There is no aftercare agency in the community to follow up with the cases of HIV-positive inmates once they are released. The Government should start such community care programmes. Also, Non-Governmental Organizations working in the field of HIV in the community may be roped in for providing aftercare services to released prisoners.

(e) Qualification of the doctors: Presently most of the Medical Doctors appointed in the prison are qualified BMS; only one doctor is an MBBS. In order to improve the quality of health services inside the prison, all the doctors appointed should at least have a MBBS degree.

Views of the Inspector General of Prisons, Maharashtra

The researcher met the Inspector General (IG) of Prisons, Maharashtra, to understand his views regarding the situation of HIV in prisons. The IG shared the following:

There were 229 Non-Governmental Organizations working in the state of Maharashtra. However, none of these NGOs were working on HIV and AIDS in the prison setting. One NGO in Mumbai was working for de-addiction of prison inmates in Mumbai Central

Prison. A liaison could be built between NGOs and the Prison Department so that NGOs working in the community on HIV and AIDS may also begin working in prison for prevention and treatment of HIV. A profile of various NGOs working in Maharashtra on HIV and AIDS could be created and depending on their credibility and scope of work, they could be invited to work inside the prison. There is a provision in the prison manual regarding premature release of terminally ill prisoners on medical grounds. Such cases are referred to the State Government by the I.G.

Commenting on the knowledge and awareness regarding HIV among prison population, the IG shared the following:

A large portion of the population are still unaware of the disease, the modes of transmission, the preventive measures and how to stay healthy if one is tested HIV positive. It is essential for each and everyone to gain knowledge about the disease, its various causes and consequences. NGOs should start making people aware and sensitive to the issue and counsel those living with HIV and AIDS. Such kind of counseling should happen on a regular and consistent basis.

Experiences and Views of the Deputy Director, National AIDS Research Institute, Pune

Since National AIDS Research Institute (NARI) is working on prevention and control of HIV and there was a liaison with Yerwada prison, the researcher had a meeting with the Deputy Director, National AIDS Research Institute (NARI), Pune. He shared that there are seven HIV clinics run by NARI which were spread across Pune district. One of these clinics was in the Department of Skin and Venereal Diseases, B. J. Medical College, and Sassoon General Hospital. Three major services were provided at the clinic:

1. HIV testing
2. Diagnosis and treatment of Sexually Transmitted Diseases (STD)
3. Advice, Guidance, and counselling for people living with HIV

Under the Antiretroviral Treatment service of the National AIDS Control Programme, NACO was providing free ART treatment (which was otherwise a very expensive treatment) in a few selected districts of Maharashtra, and Pune district was one of them.

There were two parameters for ART treatment:

1. CD4 count gets below 200
2. Viral test suggesting the requirement of ART

While discussing liaison between the prison administration and NARI, the Deputy Director mentioned that the Superintendent of Yerwada prison had requested for HIV testing of a few prisoners, the year before. The samples were sent to the clinic at NARI and were tested for HIV.

It became evident through the discussion that it was only Yerwada Jail in Pune which had approached NARI for considering cases of voluntary testing and counselling. None of the other jails had approached NARI.

Conclusion

This chapter highlights the views and experiences of the prison personnel on HIV in prison. It is evident from the above that HIV remains an issue of concern in the prison setting. One of the major findings of the present study is that prison inmates do not have easy access to health care, and in case of any illness, it is very difficult to continue the treatment. For inmates living with AIDS, continuity of treatment remains an issue due to non-availability of guards on time. This results in gap in ART and subsequent visits to the government hospital. Another important finding is that the living condition inside the prison is unhealthy, more so because of over-crowding and hence it's detrimental for the inmates living with HIV and AIDS. Prison hospitals are not well equipped to cater to the basic minimum treatment require-ments for sick inmates. The prison hospital staff are not trained on HIV and AIDS-related issues. There were hardly any NGOs working on HIV in prisons. Most of the prison personnel including the I.G. expressed keenness to involve NGOs to address the issue of HIV in prisons. Also there are no measures of HIV prevention available inside the jail.

Chapter 6
Summary and Conclusion

The main focus of this research has been to explore the experiences of prison inmates living with HIV in three jails. There are other aspects which have been taken into consideration, such as the profile of the individual inmates who are living with HIV, their socio-economic situation, their high-risk behaviour before and/or after incarceration (if any), their level of awareness and knowledge regarding HIV and AIDS, their experience in prison in terms of the prison living conditions and prison health-care facilities, any violation of ethical issues specific to their HIV status, etc. The research also attempted to capture the views of prison doctors and staff regarding the situation of HIV and AIDS in prison.

All these aspects have been covered in this research through the following objectives:

1. To examine the profile of prison inmates living with HIV.
2. To provide an in-depth analysis of the situation in which they live in prison.
3. To understand the perception of prisoners living with HIV, other prison inmates, prison personnel, and doctors (prison medical doctors and paramedical staff) regarding the prevailing health-care system in the prisons with special reference to HIV and AIDS;
4. To suggest ways and means to deal with the problems faced by prison inmates living with HIV.

In this chapter, an attempt has been made to recapitulate the main results that have emerged from the study and consider their implications. A few suggestions are also proposed for future research.

© The Author(s) 2015
S. Guin, *Prison Inmates Living with HIV in India*,
SpringerBriefs in Criminology, DOI 10.1007/978-3-319-15566-1_6

Summary of the Findings

The issue of HIV and AIDS within the closed walls of prison is often neglected as safety and security remain the prime responsibility of the prison administration. Addressing the health of prison inmates in general and those living with HIV and AIDS in particular often takes a backseat. However, a prison inmate does not cease to remain an individual inside prison and cannot be doubly punished. Public health policies meant for people living with HIV and AIDS within the general population are also equally applicable to prison inmates living with HIV and AIDS, as far as the prevention, health promotion, and care and support services are concerned. A dearth of empirical studies and knowledge regarding prison inmates living with HIV and AIDS, especially in the Indian context, makes it all the more imperative that more studies be conducted on this topic.

The present research has focused on life experiences of prison inmates living with HIV and AIDS before and after imprisonment. It is for this reason that an attempt was made to understand the lives of prison inmates living with HIV and AIDS in three prisons in the state of Maharashtra, India.

Following a qualitative approach, the study adopted a multiple-case study design to prepare detailed case studies of seven prison inmates living with HIV and AIDS through in-depth unstructured interview. Data were also gathered from the prison medical officers and the prison staff. An analysis of the data collected from the three sources—prisoners (with and without HIV), prison medical staff and prison officials—resulted in the following findings:

- Six out of the seven respondents living with HIV and AIDS fall in the age group of 25–40 years.
- Only one out of the seven respondents completed school level education.
- Three out of seven inmates were in the prison under charges of narcotics trafficking and one of them was a habitual offender.
- Four out of seven respondents had low socio-economic status.
- Four out of seven respondents were migrants from other states.
- Six out of seven respondents were not aware of HIV and AIDS before incarceration.
- None of the respondents reported to be injecting drug users.
- Four out of seven inmates contracted the disease before incarceration through high-risk sexual behaviour.
- All the seven respondents came to know of their HIV-positive status while serving their term inside the prison, when they developed opportunistic infections like skin disease and the medicine available in the prison proved ineffective.
- Overcrowding in the prisons had a direct bearing on many aspects of a prisoner's life, resulting in lack of fresh air and sunlight and leading to a deterioration of personal health and hygiene.

- Though all the seven respondents were receiving special medical diet, all of them complained about the poor quality of food and improper/inadequate nutrition.
- There are no support systems available inside the prisons to address the stress-related issues of inmates living with HIV and AIDS.
- Though all the seven respondents concurred to incidence of homosexual activity inside the prison, none of them had ever experienced or witnessed the same. However, an inmate did mention that better space was available in lieu of money or sex.
- Due to lack of infrastructure, especially equipments and supplies, only basic treatment facilities were available inside the prison hospital. Even for simple blood tests, X-RAY, and other pathological tests or treatment services, inmates were referred to the Government hospital.
- The prison hospital did not have provisions to cater to the treatment needs of inmates living with HIV. Inmates were prescribed ART when their CD4 count dropped below 200 cells/ cubic mm of blood and were provided ART at the ART centre of the Government Hospital where they were referred to by the prison doctor. Inmates were referred to the Government hospital for treatment of opportunistic infections.
- Medical examination during admission in prison was limited to recording height, weight, and identification mark.
- Referral of the sick inmates was decided by the prison doctor.
- Non-availability of guards as escorts was a major problem faced by almost all the prisoners. This led to delay, discontinuation, and inconsistency in treatment. Prisoners were transferred to the Government hospital only when they were in critical condition.
- The prison which was the referral centre for all prisons from all over Maharashtra for specialized medical treatment, was overburdened and always had the problem of limited space and manpower.
- All the four respondents who reported to have suffered from TB had undergone DOTS treatment from the respective Government hospitals.
- The prison which was not equipped with ART centre but had inmates requiring ART, were referred to the prison having an ART centre. This was a major problem for prison inmates living with HIV and AIDS, as the cumbersome process of prison transfer and non-availability of guard escorts made accessibility and continuity of medical care very difficult.
- Six of the seven prisoners were tested for HIV only when they developed opportunistic infections and were referred to the Government hospital. One of them volunteered for HIV testing out of apprehension, after developing symptoms of the disease.
- For four out of seven respondents, informed consent was taken before the test, pre- and post-test counseling was provided, and the test result was communicated by the doctor.

- Confidentiality regarding HIV-positive status could not be maintained mainly due to the special diet meant for the inmates living with HIV. In one prison, 'HIV positive' was marked on the medical files of the HIV-positive inmates. Apart from the doctor, the HIV status of the prison inmates was known to the nursing staff of the prison and the police guards who escorted them to the Government hospitals, when referred.
- Three of the inmates were ready to disclose their HIV-positive status if that helped them in getting certain advantages that might in turn help in improving their health condition.
- There was no discrimination against the prison inmate living with HIV on the grounds of their HIV-positive status. Behaviour of the police guards, prison medical doctors, and medical doctors at the Government hospitals was reported to be improper and rude towards all the inmates irrespective of their HIV status. In contrary to this, an inmate living with HIV described the doctor of one of the government hospitals as kind, someone who treated his patients well. Segregation was decided by the prison medical doctor on the basis of congeniality of the disease. Segregation was reported by one inmate from a prison who had developed skin infection; however, data could not elicit whether the skin infection was contagious.
- There were no preventive measures inside the prison against HIV and AIDS. Except for Sankalp, an NGO, which offered occasional counselling in Mumbai Central Prison, there were no NGOs working inside the prison on preventive and treatment aspects of HIV. Pune District AIDS Control Society had started voluntary counselling and testing centre inside the Yerwada prison.
- A thorough examination of the Prison Visitors Book revealed that there were no particular comments by the prison visitors regarding the health of the inmates.
- The prison doctors did not receive any training on HIV and AIDS and human rights of prisoners, before they were appointed at the prison.
- Lack of lab technician, insufficient number of prison medical doctors, and inadequate medical equipments and supplies within the prison were highlighted as the major shortcomings inside the prison.

Conclusion

In conclusion, it can be stated that through this study, the experiences of prison inmates living with HIV were explored against the backdrop of prison living conditions and the health-care services inside the prison. It has emerged that prison living conditions are not conducive for the health of prison inmates living with HIV and the medical facilities and services available for HIV-positive prison inmates are inadequate, difficult to access, and in some cases absent. The prison environment itself poses particular health risks. Inside the prison, the inmates are deprived of their liberty and are fully dependent on the state authority. The state has a greater obligation to provide the necessary health care to the prisoners, as they are citizens who have been confined by the State, restricting their access to services available within the community. The availability of treatment for AIDS in prisons, including the essential medicines, is based on the general principle that the level of heath care in prisons should be at least equivalent to that in the outside community.

Recommendations

The following major suggestions have emerged from the study to facilitate better access to improved health care for prisoners living with HIV and AIDS:

Facilitating Treatment, Care, and Support to Inmates Living with HIV and AIDS

- Diagnosis and treatment in the context of HIV and AIDS are often complex. So, health-care services in the prison should include physicians specialized in HIV and AIDS, on a regular or weekly basis. They may even encourage voluntary HIV testing, followed by the required treatment. The prison health-care services should collaborate with the Maharashtra State AIDS Control Society, the respective District AIDS Control Societies, and the major private hospitals to facilitate optimal health care of prison inmates living with HIV and AIDS.
- Importance should be given to pre-test and post-test counseling.
- Once an inmate is tested HIV positive, the prison authorities should make efforts to ensure that the wife and children of the inmates are also tested for HIV through informed consent.
- Department of Prisons should collaborate with the Medical universities to encourage medical students to take up assignments on various issues associated with HIV and AIDS inside prisons.
- Prisoners who require ART from J.J. Hospital, Mumbai, should be transferred to prisons other than Mumbai Central Prison, which are located near Mumbai like Thane Central Prison. This will help to deal with the overcrowding at Mumbai Central Prison and ensure inmates receive continued treatment without any gap.
- The special division of the police department for prisons, which presently monitors the provision of police guards round the clock at the prisons, may be strengthened to provide guards exclusively meant for medical services for the prison inmates, so as to facilitate the provision of guard escorts for inmates to the Government hospitals.

- Strengthening of the already existing prison visiting system[1] can play an important role in addressing the moral, psychological, and social needs of the prison inmates living with HIV and AIDS. The Prison Department should make efforts to facilitate the access of inmates with their family members or friends.
- Health Inspectors appointed by the Directorate of Health Services should visit the prison at regular intervals and check the living conditions of the prison. A thorough check of the prison meals has to be done by the health department to assess the calorific value of the special medical diet provided to the HIV-positive prisoners.
- Other alternative medicines like Homeopathy, Unani, and Ayurveda should be encouraged in prisons to provide medical care to the inmates. This will in some cases be economical and effective and will never depend on the availability of guards.
- Care has to be taken in case of any of the contagious diseases like TB, malaria, diarrhoea, respiratory problems, and skin diseases. Periodic surveillance should be made to monitor such diseases among inmates in prison.
- Prison transfer of HIV-positive inmates who are migrants should be given priority. This issue should be discussed at annual meetings organized by the Bureau of Police Research and Development (BPR&D), for the Deputy General of Police (Prison) and Inspector General of Police (Prison), so that the process of prison transfer becomes easier and quicker.
- A thorough monitoring system for health care in prisons has to be established where prison visitors appointed by the National Human Rights Commission should visit the prison at regular intervals and listen to the grievances of the prisoners and take necessary action.
- At the time of admission to the prison, prisoners should be provided with information related to HIV and AIDS and a list of NGOs (which have collaboration with the Department of Prison) which will visit the prison at regular intervals to provide various support services. The list might be given to the inmates at the time of release so that the prisoner may contact the NGO (s) post release.
- Each inmate should be provided with detailed information regarding HIV and AIDS.
- Prisoners who are willing to share information and knowledge regarding HIV and AIDS inside the jail should be encouraged and trained to become peer educators.
- Various legal provisions (for example the Code of Criminal Procedure Amendment Act 2005 which came into effect on July 2006) may be implemented to release certain categories of inmates, mainly the undertrial prisoners who are most often charged with petty offences. This will help to decongest the jail and thus minimize the problem of overcrowding. This will have positive health impact on the prisoners. Moreover, this will eventually help in the provision of proper care, treatment, and support to the HIV-positive inmates.

---

[1] Subsection (25), section 59 of The Prisons Act of 1894, empowers State to make rules for the appointment and guidance of official and non-official visitors to the prisons.

- Availability of condoms: A policy to distribute condoms in prisons is often controversial because government officials do not wish to discuss homosexual activity in prisons and a good portion deny even the incidence of any such. In a society where sex is considered a taboo and homosexual activity a crime, provision of condoms for homosexual activity in prisons is a topic which can never be considered fit for parliamentary debate. Nevertheless, condoms may be made available in the prison and should also be distributed when the HIV-positive inmate is released either on furlough or after serving the prison tenure.
- At the time of release of the inmates living with HIV and AIDS, either on furlough or after serving their term, proper counselling should be provided to them and their family.

Involvement of NGOs and Other Institutions Working on HIV

Help from the NGOs may be sought to enhance the HIV and AIDS care and treatment in a holistic way.

- *For palliative care of HIV and AIDS inmates*: Palliative care is holistic, aiming for the physical, psychological, social, and spiritual well-being of the patient and his/her family (Bollini & Gunchenko 2001). Thus, cooperation and collaboration with the community-based organizations should be sought in order to provide palliative care to HIV and AIDS inmates during their stay in prison as well as when they are released.
- *For counseling, testing, and treatment*: Non-Governmental Organizations should be encouraged to work in the prisons on HIV and AIDS. These NGOs may carry out pre-test and post-test counseling, provide with testing facilities, and carry out the required treatment on a regular basis. Efforts should be made by the prison department to identify such NGOs which are already working in the community on HIV and AIDS and having a consistent and substantive track record of effective programme implementation, to work inside the prison on HIV and AIDS.
- *Liaison with NARI for HIV testing inside prison*: The National AIDS Research Institute located in Pune used to test blood samples of prison inmates from Yerwada Central Prison. NARI was open for any kind of liaison including testing inside the prison.
- *For awareness generation to prevent HIV-related TB*: For prevention of TB, raising awareness on TB can enhance early case detection and prompt initiation of treatment. The awareness generation may include information on the modes of transmission of TB, its symptoms, treatment, available TB services and access, and means of reducing risks of infection. All prisoners and prison staff should be aware of the importance of early detection and complete and continued treatment of TB. Regular film shows on HIV and AIDS awareness and education followed by interactive sessions should be organized at regular intervals, particularly at the time of admission of the prisoner and at the time of release.

Arrangements must also be made to invite the family members of inmates to participate in such shows.

- *Complimentary copies of various health magazines* with information on HIV and AIDS may be distributed to the prison department. The articles on HIV and AIDS may then be translated in local language and made available along with the newspapers inside the prison.

Compassionate Release of Terminally Ill Prisoners

AIDS is a terminal illness as death can be averted or delayed only with the triple drug antiretroviral regimens. In the absence of such treatments or in the absence of optimal treatments for the opportunistic illnesses associated with AIDS, the life expectancy of the patient gets drastically reduced. Such patients should be considered terminally ill (Bollini & Gunchenko 2001). These terminally ill inmates should be considered for compassionate early release from the prison. Prisoners on the verge of death should be released. Pre-release programmes for HIV and AIDS inmates should be encouraged. WHO guidelines advocate early release of prisoners in the advanced stages of AIDS. The motivation behind a policy of early release is to allow a person to die in dignity, either in their own home or with their family, rather than forcing them to die in isolation and alone inside the confined walls of the prison.

Prevention of HIV-Related TB Disease

The spread of TB in prisons can be prevented through early detection of individual cases and making treatment accessible for all those inmates diagnosed with TB. Prison administration may collaborate with the TB services in the Government hospital and make arrangements for regular checkups for TB inside the prison. This will also ensure the continuity of treatment and appropriate medical follow-up when individuals with TB are arrested or released from prison.

Suggestions for Further Research

Three broad areas for further research on HIV and AIDS in prisons are outlined below:

- Epidemiological research on the prevalence of HIV and AIDS in prisons in India to know the exact data on the number of prison inmates living with HIV and AIDS.

- An extensive survey research of the health-care scenario with particular reference to HIV and AIDS in all prisons in India to understand the gaps in access to health care in prison for prison inmates living with HIV and AIDS.
- A comprehensive study on the knowledge, awareness, and attitude of prison inmates and prison staff on HIV and AIDS to devise a policy framework for addressing the issue of HIV and AIDS in Indian prisons.

References

Aggarwal, A., Arora, U., & Nagpal, N. (2005). Seroprevalence of HIV in Central Jail Inmates of Amritsar. *Indian Journal of Community Medicine, 30*(4), 151.

Asl, R. T., Eshrati, B., Dell, C. A., Taylor, K., Afshar, P., Kamali, M., et al. (2013). Outcome assessment of a triangular clinic as a harm reduction intervention in Rajaee-Shahr Prison, Iran. *Harm Reduction Journal, 10*(41), 1–11. doi:10.1186/1477-7517-10-41.

Bedi, K. (2002). *It's always possible*. New Delhi: Sterling Publishers Private Limited.

Betteridge, G. (2004). Prisoners' health and human rights in the HIV/AIDS epidemic. *HIV/AIDS Policy and law review, 9*(3), 96–99. Retrieved October 28, 2014, from http://www.aidslaw.ca/publications/interfaces/downloadFile.php?ref=177.

Blogg, S., Utomo, B., Silitonga, N., Hidayati, D. A. N., & Sattler, G. (2014). Indonesian national inmate Bio-Behavioral Survey for HIV and Syphilis prevalence and risk behaviors in Prisons and Detention Centers, 2010. *SAGE Open, 2014*(January–March), 1–7. doi:10.1177/2158244013518924.

Bollini, P., & Gunchenko, A. (2001). Treatment of HIV/AIDS. In P. Bollini (Ed.), *HIV in prisons: A reader with particular reference to the newly independent states* (pp. 67–146). Europe: World Health Organization. Retrieved October 28, 2014, from http://www.euro.who.int/__data/assets/pdf_file/0008/78551/E77016.pdf.

Braithwaite, R. L., Hammett, T. M., & Mayberry, R. M. (1996). *Prisons and AIDS: A public health challenge*. CA: Jossey-Bass Inc.

Bryan, A., Robbins, R. N., Ruiz, M. S., & O'Neill, D. (2006). Effectiveness of an HIV prevention intervention in prison among African Americans, Hispanics, and Caucasians. *Health Education & Behavior, 33*(2), 154–177.

Bureau of Police Research and Development. (2003). *Model Prison Manual for the Superintendent and Management of Prisons in India*. New Delhi: Ministry of Home Affairs, Government of India.

Burris, S., & Villena, D. (2004). Adapting to the reality of HIV- Difficult policy choices in Russia, China, and India. *Human Rights, 31*(4), 10–14. Retrieved September 30, 2008, from, http://www.abanet.org/irr/hr/fall04/reality.htm.

Burstein, J. Q. (1977). *Conjugal visits in prisons: Psychological and social consequences*. Toronto: Lexington Books.

Carelse, M. (1994). *AIDS prevention and high risk behaviour in juvenile correctional institutions*. Bellville: University of Western Cape.

© The Author(s) 2015
S. Guin, *Prison Inmates Living with HIV in India*,
SpringerBriefs in Criminology, DOI 10.1007/978-3-319-15566-1

Castro, K. G., Ward, J. W., Slutsker, L., Buehler, J. W., Jaffe, H. W., Berkelman, R. L., et al. (1992). Revised classification system for HIV infection and expanded surveillance case definition for AIDS among adolescents and adults. *CDC prevention guidelines database*. Retrieved October 28, 2014, from http://wonder.cdc.gov/wonder/prevguid/m0018871/m0018871.asp

Census of India. (2011). Retrieved October 28, 2014, from http://censusindia.gov.in/

Chakrapani, V., Kamei, R., Kipgen, H., & Kumar, J. (2013). Access to harm reduction and HIV-related treatment services inside Indian prisons: Experiences of formerly incarcerated injecting drug users. *International Journal of Prisoner Health, 9*(2), 82–91.

Chattoraj, B. N. (2006). *Children of women prisoners in Indian jail*. Delhi: LNJN National Institute of Criminology and Forensic Sciences.

CHRI. (2008). *Community participation in prison, A civil society perspective*. New Delhi: Commonwealth Human Rights Initiative. Retrieved September 12, 2014, from http://www.humanrightsinitiative.org/publications/prisons/community_participation_in_prisons.pdf.

Collica, K. (2002). Levels of knowledge of risk perceptions about HIV/AIDS among female inmates in New York state: Can prison-based HIV programs set the stage for behavior change? *The Prison Journal, 82*(1), 101–124.

Cusack, L., & Singh, S. (1994). *HIV and AIDS care: Practical approaches*. London: Chapman and Hall.

Dara, M., Grzemska, M., Kimerling, M. E., Reyes, H., Zagorskiy, A. (2009). *Guidelines for control of tuberculosis in prisons*. USAID, TBCTA, ICRC. Retrieved September 11, 2014, from http://pdf.usaid.gov/pdf_docs/PNADP462.pdf.

Dickson, D. T. (2001). *HIV, AIDS, and the law: Legal issues for social work practice and policy*. New York: Walter de Gruyter Inc.

Dolan, K., Kite, B., Black, E., Aceijas, C., & Stimson, G. V. (2007). HIV in prison in low-income and middle-income countries. *The Lancet Infectious Diseases, 7*(1), 32–41.

Dolan, K., & Larney, S. (2010). HIV in Indian prisons: Risk behaviour, prevalence, prevention and treatment. *Indian Journal of Medical Research, 132*(6), 696–700.

Dolan, K., Lowe, D., & Shearer, J. (2004). Evaluation of the condom distribution program in New South Wales prisons, Australia. *Journal of Law, Medicine & Ethics, 32*, 124–128.

Donde, S. (2006, August). *HIV risk behaviour in prisons among drug users in Mumbai*. Paper presented at XVI International AIDS Conference, Toronto, Canada.

Fox, V. (1983). *Correctional institutions*. Englewood Cliffs, NJ: Prentice-Hall.

Gillespie, W. (2005). A multilevel model of drug abuse inside prison. *The Prison Journal, 85*, 223–246.

Glaser, J. B., & Greifinger, R. B. (1993). Correctional health care: A public health opportunity (Review). *Annals of Internal Medicine, 118*(2), 139–145.

Goffman, E. (1961). *Asylums: Essays on the social situations of mental patients and other inmates*. Chicago: Aldine Publishing Company.

Government of India. (2007). *Report of the Committee on Draft National Policy on Criminal Justice*. New Delhi: Ministry of Home Affairs.

Goyer, K. C. (2003). *HIV/Aids in prison, problems, policies and potential, Monograph No 79*, Institute for Security Studies. Retrieved September 5, 2014, from http://www.issafrica.org/publications/monographs/monograph-79-hivaids-in-prison-problems-policies-and-potential-kc-goyer.

Grinstead, O. A., Zack, B., & Faigeles, B. (1999). Collaborative research to prevent HIV among male prison inmates and their female partners. *Health Education & Behavior, 26*(2), 225–238.

Guin, S. (2007, February). *Right to health of prisoners in India*. Paper presented at the 1st International and 30th All India Criminology Conference of the Indian Society of Criminology (ISC) organized by the Indian Criminological Congress, University of Calcutta, West Bengal.

Haghdoost, A., Mirzazadeh, A., Shokoohi, M., Sedaghat, A., & Gouya, M. M. (2013). HIV trend among Iranian prisoners in 1990s and 2000s; analysis of aggregated data from HIV sentinel sero-surveys. *Harm Reduction Journal., 10*(32), 2–5.

Haikerwal, B. S. (1939). *Social aspects of crime in India*. London: MacMillian.

HIV/AIDS among Youth. (2008). *CDC HIV/AIDS fact sheet*. Retrieved July 19, 2014, from http://www.cdc.gov/hiv/resources/factsheets/PDF/youth.pdf

Hudson, A. L., Nyamathi, A., Bhattacharya, D., Marlow, E., Shoptaw, S., Marfisee, M., et al. (2011). Impact of prison status on HIV-related risk behaviors. *AIDS Behaviour, 15*(2), 340–346.

Inciardi, J. A., Surratt, H. L., Martin, S. S., O'Connell, D. J., Salandy, A. D., & Beard, R. A. (2007). Developing a multimedia HIV and hepatitis intervention for drug involved offenders reentering the community. *The Prison Journal, 87*(1), 111–142.

Inspector General of Prisons. (2006). *Handbook of prison statistics 2004–2005*. Pune: Author.

International Institute of Population Sciences (IIPS) & Macro International. (2007). *National Family Health Survey (NFHS-3), 2005–2006: India* (Vol. 1). Mumbai: Author.

Jaiswal, T. B. L. (1992). *AIDS: Causes and prevention*. New Delhi: Mittal Publications.

Jurgens, R. (2007). *Evidence for action technical papers. Effectiveness of intervention to address HIV in prisons*. Geneva: World Health Organization. Retrieved September 10, 2014, from http://whqlibdoc.who.int/publications/2007/9789241596190_eng.pdf.

Kakar, D. N. (1994). *AIDS prevention: The emerging challenge*. Haryana: The Environment Society of Haryana.

Kalantar, T., & Alijev, L. (2005). An HIV intervention: The work of the Convictus Eesti group in Estonian prisons. *International Journal of Prisoner Health, 1*(2), 283–285.

Karnam, M. (2009). Deaths in prisons in Andhra Pradesh. *Economic and Political Weekly, 44*(11), 19–23.

Khan, M. Z. (1990). *Work by jail inmates*. New Delhi: Inter-India Publications.

Klein, S. J., Gieryic, S. M., O'Connell, D. A., Hall, J. Y., & Klopf, L. C. (2002). Availability of HIV prevention services within New York state correctional facilities during 1999–2000: Results of a survey. *The Prison Journal, 82*(1), 69–83.

Krebs, C. P. (2002). High-risk HIV transmission behaviour in prison and the prison subculture. *The Prison Journal, 82*(1), 19–49.

Krishnan, J. K. (2003). The rights of the new untouchables: A constitutional analysis of HIV Jurisprudence in India. *Human Rights Quarterly, 25*(3), 791–819.

Laufer, F. N., Arriola, K. R. J., Dawson-rose, C. S., Kumaravelu, K., & Rapposelli, K. K. (2002). From jail to community: Innovative strategies to enhance continuity of HIV/AIDS care. *The Prison Journal, 82*(1), 84–100.

Lawyers Collective HIV/AIDS Unit. (2008). *National coalition meeting on the HIV/AIDS bill*. New Delhi: Lawyers Collective HIV/AIDS Unit. Retrieved September 3, 2008, from http://www.lawyerscollective.org/hiv-coalition.

Lines, R., & Stover, H. (2005). *HIV/AIDS prevention, care, treatment, and support in prison settings: A framework for an effective national response*. New York: UNODC, WHO, UNAIDS.

Macalino, G. E., Hou, J. C., Kumar, M. S., Taylor, L. E., Sumantera, I. G., & Rich, J. D. (2004). Hepatitis C infection and incarcerated population. *International Journal of Drug Policy, 15*(2), 103–114.

Madhurima. (2009). *Women, crime and prison life*. New Delhi: Deep & Deep Publications Pvt. Ltd.

Mahapatra, D. (2013, December 12). Supreme Court makes homosexuality a crime again. *The Times of India*. Retrieved August 23, 2014, from http://timesofindia.indiatimes.com/india/Supreme-Court-makes-homosexuality-a-crime-again/articleshow/27230690.cms.

Mehta, S., & Sodhi, S. K. (2004). *Understanding AIDS: Myths, efforts and achievements*. New Delhi: APH.

Mullings, J. L., Marquart, J. W., & Hartley, D. J. (2003). Exploring the effects of childhood sexual abuse and its impact on HIV/AIDS risk-taking behavior among women prisoners. *The Prison Journal, 83*(4), 442–463.

NACO. (2008). *HIV sentinel surveillance round 2008: National action plan September 2008—June 2009*. Delhi: Ministry of Health and Family Welfare, Government of India.

Nag, A., Chattopadhayay, D., Nag, S., Saha, G., VIHC JAILAIDS Group. (2006, August). *Prevalence of STDs/HIV infection in prisons of West Bengal and prevention programs in India.* Paper presented at XVI International AIDS Conference Toronto, Toronto, Canada.

Nagaraj, S. G., Sarvade, M., Muthanna, L., Raju, R., Aju, S., Sarvade N. M. (2000, July). *HIV seroprevalance and prevalent attitudes amongst the prisoners: A case study in Mysore, Karnataka state India.* Paper presented at the XIII International AIDS Conference, Durban.

National Aids Control Organization. (2013). *HIV Sentinel Surveillance 2012–13. A Technical Brief.* New Delhi: Ministry of Health & Family Welfare. Retrieved September 30, 2014, from www.naco.gov.in.

National Crime Records Bureau. (2012). *Crime in India 2011.* New Delhi: Ministry of Home Affairs.

National Human Rights Commission. (2006). *Annual report 2004–05.* New Delhi: Author.

Naz Foundation files Curative Petition challenging the Supreme Court judgment on Section 377. (2014). Retrieved October 15, 2014, from http://www.lawyerscollective.org/updates/naz-foundation-files-curative-petition-challenging-supreme-court-judgment-section-377.html.

OHCHR. (1996–2004). *Introduction to HIV/AIDS and human rights.* Office of the High Commissioner for Human Rights United Nations Office at Geneva. Retrieved December 19, 2005, from http://www.ohchr.org/english/issues/hiv/introhiv.htm.

Oppong, J. R., Kutch, L., Tiwari, C., & Arbona, S. (2013). Vulnerable places: Prison locations, socioeconomic status, and HIV infection in Texas. *The Professional Geographer, 66*(4), 653–663. doi:10.1080/00330124.2013.852040.

Pal, B., Acharya, A., & Satyanarayana, K. (1999). Seroprevalence of HIV infection among jail inmates in Orissa. *Indian Journal of Medical Research, 109*, 199–201.

Palaniappan K. (1995). *Trend of HIV among STD patients, pregnant women and truckers through unlinked anonymous screening in India.* Paper presented at 3rd International Conference in AIDS in Asia and the Pacific 1995, Chiang Mai, Thailand.

Palve, A., Borges, N., Asfar, S., Pandit, D. (2006, August). *Prison employees and inmates, workplace intervention program for risk reduction in prisons.* Paper presented at XVI International AIDS Conference, Toronto, Canada.

Pavri, K. M. (1992). *Challenge of AIDS.* New Delhi: National Book Trust.

Plumber, M. & Pathak, M. K. (2011, April 19). Time to free Mumbai of its overcrowded prison? *DNA India.* Retrieved May 25, 2014.

Raghavan, V., & Nair, R. (2011). *A study of the socio economic profile and rehabilitation needs of Muslim community in prisons in Maharashtra.* Unpublished report, TISS, Mumbai.

Ray, R. (2002). *Drug abuse among prison population: A case study of Tihar Jail.* National Survey on Extent, Pattern, and Trends of Drug Abuse in India, Ministry of Social Justice and Empowerment, Government of India and United Nations International Drug Control Programme, Regional Office for South Asia, Delhi.

Richards, E. P. (1999). HIV: Testing, screening, and confidentiality—An American Perspective. In R. Bennett & C. A. Erin (Eds.). *HIV and AIDS, testing, screening and confidentiality.* Oxford: Oxford University Press. Retrieved October 28, 2014, from http://biotech.law.lsu.edu/cphl/articles/american-hiv.htm

Saini, M. (2008, July 17). Five Jail wheat Samples Failed Test. *The Times of India.*

Saprem (n. d.). Pinjra Project. Retrieved December 22, 2008, from http://www.sapremngo.org/pinjra_project.htm.

Sarangi, J. (1999, September 22–25). *Tihar prisons: A correctional experiment.* Paper presented at VIII International Symposium on Torture- A challenge to the health, legal and other professions, organised by the NHRC and IRCT at New Delhi.

Schrag, C. (1961). Leadership among prison inmates. *American Sociological Review, 19*, 37–42.

Shaikh, A. (2010, August 17). Murder convict escapes from Yerawada prison. *The Times of India.* Mumbai.

Shalihu, N., Pretorius, L., Dyk, A., Stoep, A. V., & Hagopian, A. (2014). Namibian prisoners describe barriers to HIV antiretroviral therapy adherence. *AIDS Care, 26*, 968–75. doi:10.108 0/09540121.2014.880398.

Shankardass, R. D. (2000). *Punishment and the prison—Indian and international perspectives*. New Delhi: Sage Publications.

Sifunda, S., Reddy, P. S., Braithwaite, R. B., Stephens, T., Bhengu, S., Ruiter, R. A. C., et al. (2007). The relationship between alcohol and drug use and sexual behaviour amongst prison inmates in developing countries. The case of South Africa. *International Journal of Prisoner Health, 3*(1), 3–15.

Sifunda, S., Reddy, P. S., Braithwaite, R., Stephens, T., Bhengu, S., Ruiter, R. A. C., et al. (2008). The effectiveness of a peer-led HIV/AIDS and STI health education intervention for prison inmates in South Africa. *Health Education & Behavior, 35*(4), 494–508.

Simooya, O., & Sanjobo, N. (2001). 'In but free': An HIV/AIDS intervention in an African prison. *Culture, Health & Sexuality, 3*(2), 241–251.

Singh, M. (2007). HIV/AIDS. *From the Lawyers Collective, 22*(8), 25–30.

Singh, S. (2008). Prison inmate awareness of HIV and AIDS in Durban, South Africa. *Sociological Bulletin, 57*(2), 193–210.

Singh, S., Prasad, R., & Mohanty, A. (1999). High prevalence of sexually transmitted and blood-borne infections amongst the inmates of a district jail in Northern India. *International Journal of STD & AIDS, 10*, 475–478.

Somasundaram, P. M., & Sundar, S. (1997). Aiding AIDS prisoners: Issues and options. *The Indian Journal of Criminology, 25*(2), 61–69.

Sonawane, S. (2014, April 15). Plans to train inmates of Nashik jail in honey, silk cultivation. *The Times of India*. Mumbai.

Srivastava, S. P. (1977). *The Indian prison community*. Lucknow: Pustak Kendra.

Stubblefield, E., & Wohl, D. (2000). Prisons and jails worldwide: Update from the 13th International Conference on AIDS. *HEPP News, 3*, 1–3.

Sundar, M., Ravikumar, K. K., & Sudarshan, M. K. A. (1995). Cross-sectional seroprevalence survey for HIV-1 and high risk sexual behaviour of seropositives in a prison in India. *Indian Journal of Public Health, 39*(3), 116–118.

Swartz, J. A., Lurigio, A. J., & Weiner, D. A. (2004). Correlates of HIV-risk behaviors among prison inmates: Implications for tailored Aids prevention programming. *The Prison Journal, 84*(4), 486–504.

Sykes, G. M. (1958). *The Society of Captives: A study of a maximum security prison*. Princeton, NJ: Princeton University Press.

The Dublin Declaration on HIV/AIDS in Prisons in Europe and Central Asia. (2005). *International Journal of Prisoner Health, 1*(1), 91–98.

Thomas, G. (1994). *AIDS in India, myth and reality*. News Delhi: Rawat Publications.

Thomas, C. W., & Cage, R. J. (1977). Correlates of prison drug use: An evaluation of two conceptual models. *Criminology, 15*, 193–210.

Tiwari, A. (2002). *Medical facilities in Indian prisons: Role of prison doctors and para-medical staff to uphold the right to health of prisoners*. Mumbai: Tata Institute of Social Sciences.

Tiwari, A. (2006). Premature release of prisoners in India: A human rights perspective. *The Indian Journal of Criminology & Criminalistics, XXVII*(1), 11–24.

UNAIDS. (1997). *Prisons and AIDS: UNAIDS technical update*. Geneva: UNAIDS. Retrieved October 10, 2014, from https://www.unodc.org/documents/hiv-aids/UNAIDS%20prison%20 and%20AIDS.pdf.

UNAIDS. (1999). *WHO guidelines on HIV infection and AIDS in prison*. Geneva: UNAIDS. Retrieved September 16, 2014, from http://www.who.int/hiv/pub/idu/guidelines_hiv_prisons/en/

UNAIDS. (2002). *Summary of the Declaration of Commitment on HIV/AIDS, United Nations General Assembly Special Session on HIV/AIDS, 25–27 June 2001*. New York: UNAIDS. Retrieved October 15, 2014, from http://www.unaids.org/en/media/unaids/contentassets/dataimport/pub/report/2002/jc668-keepingpromise_en.pdf

UNAIDS. (2004). *Report on the Global AIDS Epidemic, UNAIDS Fourth Global Report, 2004*. Switzerland: UNAIDS. Retrieved December 12, 2005, from http://www.unaids.org.

UNAIDS. (2006). *International guidelines on HIV/AIDS and Human Rights 2006 consolidated version*. Geneva: UNAIDS. Retrieved February 28, 2015, from http://www.ohchr.org/Documents/Publications/HIVAIDSGuidelinesen.pdf.

UNAIDS. (2013). *Global Report. UNAIDS report on the global AIDS epidemic 2013*. New York: UNAIDS. Retrieved September 12, 2014, from http://www.unaids.org/en/media/unaids/contentassets/documents/epidemiology/2013/gr2013/UNAIDS_Global_Report_2013_en.pdf.

UNAIDS. (n.d.). *UNAIDS policy brief: HIV, food security and nutrition*. Available from www.unaids.org/en/.../jc1565_policy_brief_nutrition_long_en.pdf [Accessed 14/05/2014]

UNODC. (2002). *The extent, patterns and trends of drug abuse in India: National Survey*. New Delhi: UNODC.

UNODC. (2006). Report of the *National training programme to address HIV prevention amongst incarcerated substance users*. Organized by the United National Office on Drugs and Crime (UNODC) Regional Office for South Asia, New Delhi, in collaboration with Tata Institute of Social Sciences, Mumbai from February 27 to March 3, 2006.

UNODC. (2007). *Module for prison intervention: South Asia, preventing drug use among incarcerated substance users*. India: United Nations Office on Drugs and Crime, Regional Office for South Asia.

Weilandt, C., Stöver, H., Eckert, J., & Grigoryan, G. (2007). Anonymous survey on infectious diseases and related risk behaviour among Armenian prisoners and prison staff. *International Journal of Prisoner Health, 3*(1), 17–28.

West, A. D. (2001). HIV/AIDS education for Latina inmates: The delimiting impact of culture on prevention efforts. *The Prison Journal, 81*(1), 20–41.

WHO, UNODC, UNAIDS. (2008). *HIV and AIDS in places of detention: A toolkit for policymakers, programme managers, prison officers and health care providers in prison settings*. Vienna: UNODC. Available at www.unodc.org/unodc/en/hiv-aids/publications.html.

Williams, J. R. (2008). The Declaration of Helsinki and public health. *Bulletin of the World Health Organization, 86*, 650–651.

World Health Organization. (2014). *Prisons and health*. Geneva: WHO. Retrieved September 11, 2014, from http://www.euro.who.int/__data/assets/pdf_file/0005/249188/Prisons-and-Health.pdf

Yin, R. K. (2009). *Case study research: Design and methods*. Los Angeles: Sage.

Zeichner, S. L., & Read, J. S. (2006). *Handbook of pediatric HIV care*. Cambridge, UK: Cambridge University Press.

Index

© The Author(s) 2015
S. Guin, *Prison Inmates Living with HIV in India*,
SpringerBriefs in Criminology, DOI 10.1007/978-3-319-15566-1

Printed in the United States
By Bookmasters